ACUPRESSURE
TECHNIQUES

ACUPRESSURE TECHNIQUES

A SELF-HELP GUIDE

JULIAN KENYON, M.D.

Healing Arts Press
Rochester, Vermont

Healing Arts Press
One Park Street
Rochester, Vermont 05767
Web Site: http://www.gotoit.com

Note to the reader: This book is intended as an informational guide. The remedies, approaches, and techniques described herein are meant to supplement, and not to be a substitute for, professional medical care or treatment. They should not be used to treat a serious ailment without prior consultation with a qualified healthcare professional.

Library of Congress Cataloging-in-Publication Data

Kenyon, J. N. (Julian, N.)
    Acupressure techniques, a self-help guide.
    Bibliography: p.
    Includes index.
    1. Acupressure. 2. Self-care, Health. I. Title.
RM723.A27K46 1988   615.8'22 88-30105
ISBN 0-89281-280-X original
ISBN 0-89281-641-4 reissue

Printed and bound in the United States

10 9 8 7 6 5 4 3 2 1

Healing Arts Press is a division of Inner Traditions International

Distributed to the book trade in Canada by Publishers Group West (PGW), Toronto, Ontario

Distributed to the health food trade in Canada by Alive Books, Toronto and Vancouver

CONTENTS

To Rachel J.

HOW TO USE THIS BOOK

This manual is for home use and centres around deep finger pressure over acupuncture points. The direction of finger pressure massage is of great importance, as the acupuncture meridian system has a directional flow. Therefore the points should be massaged in the correct direction. This is clearly indicated on all the charts accompanying each condition.

Deep pressure with the thumb is the best way of stimulating acupuncture points. **Above all, remember to use deep firm pressure, preferably with the thumb. If acupressure is not uncomfortable to begin with then the pressure on the point should be increased until some discomfort is felt. This initial discomfort will soon pass off.**

The stimulation of the point Large Intestine 4 is shown in *Figure 1*.

Note that the direction of massage is up towards the wrist with strong movements in this direction and less strong motion in the opposite direction. The point should be massaged for a number of minutes until a deep, achey, numbing feeling is produced. Make sure to search around carefully for the point, and often you will find that it is slightly tender to deep pressure. Very sensitive people will respond to light massage, although the majority of people require firm, deep pressure with a thumb over the appropriate energy point.

Each point should be massaged in turn according to the instructions for each condition. An average acupressure session may last anything up to 20 minutes. It is entirely possible to carry out acupressure on yourself, but it is significantly more effective if you can get a friend or relative to do it for you. If the points hurt a bit at first on deep pressure, try to persist as eventually this tenderness will disappear entirely. If you are able to tolerate some mild

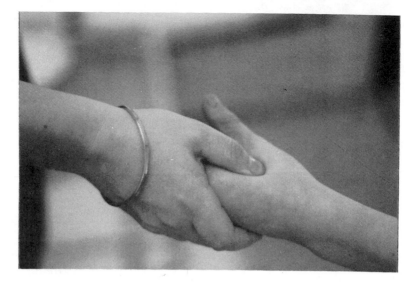

Figure 1. Acupressure stimulation of Large Intestine 4 energy point.

discomfort in the early part of each acupressure session, the results will be that much better.

Acupressure stimulation of ear points is of some importance, and is best done with a blunt object such as a matchstick, although a finger nail can be used. *Figures 2 and 3* show energy points being stimulated on the ear.

It is particularly important, in the case of the ear, to search round very carefully with the thumb nail for a period of some 2 or 3 minutes until a tender point has been located. Invariably the right point on the ear will be slightly tender. If it is not, then it is almost certain that you have chosen the wrong point. Absolute accuracy with point location is essential on the ear. Asking someone else to carry out ear acupressure on you is a decided advantage since it is much easier for another person to carry it out.

The purpose of this book is two-fold. Firstly, it aims to give some scientific backing as to how acupressure can help a wide number of conditions. Secondly, it will explain the treatment of approximately thirty common pain problems and thirty other minor conditions.

In most *chronic* (long-standing, or lasting longer than 2 weeks) conditions a number of treatments will be required, possibly as many as twenty. In most *acute* conditions (which have only been present for a short time – less than 2 weeks) fewer treatments are

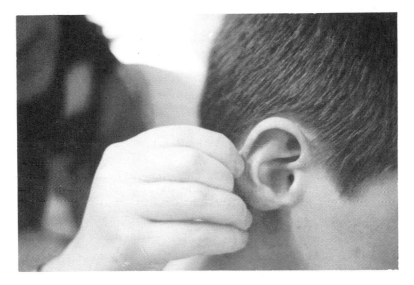

Figure 2. Acupressure stimulation of an ear energy point using a finger nail.

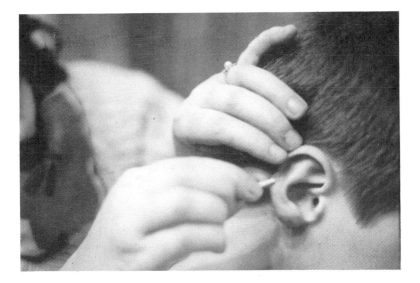

Figure 3. Acupressure stimulation of an ear energy point using a matchstick.

required, in many cases only one.

Look up the condition you wish to treat by consulting the index at the back of the book. This will give you the relevant page to look up and show you the points to use. Treat each point for 2–3 minutes, or for as long as it takes to produce a deep, achey, numbing type of feeling over the point. Repeat the treatment daily until some benefit is obtained. As you begin to improve then extend the time between each treatment.

If your condition does not respond, consult a doctor (a list of addresses of recognized medical organizations with a practical working knowledge of acupuncture in different countries is given on page 215. It is likely that doctors with this experience would be the best ones to advise you). One of the main points you may need advice about is whether a treatment approach using acupressure is appropriate for your condition, which in some cases it will not be.

If you have more than a passing interest in acupuncture, and want to know what the present theories are and how the treatment works, then the sections before the treatment for specific conditions section will be of interest to you. For the real enthusiast, some suggestions for further reading are listed on page 213.

This book and the information contained in it in no way constitutes a licence or invitation to set up as a practitioner of any kind. It is merely a simple and interesting guide to self-treatment for a number of common ailments, using acupressure.

TRADITIONAL ACUPUNCTURE THEORY

Acupressure makes use of the system of acupuncture for its success. Therefore a brief introduction to acupuncture is necessary in order to fully understand how and where to use acupressure with confidence and absolute safety.

Acupuncture is a very ancient system of treatment, and is part of the discipline of traditional Chinese medicine. This embraces many other systems of healing, quite apart from acupuncture, such as traditional Chinese herbal medicine. Acupuncture is therefore not, and never has been, a complete system of medicine in its own right. It is nevertheless dramatically effective in many conditions which often have not responded to conventional approaches. Acupuncture's main use is in treating chronic painful conditions, which, after dental caries (tooth decay) and the common cold, are the most common afflictions of the human race. Its effectiveness has enabled acupuncture to survive against enormous odds at times. It was banned by law in China at the beginning of this century, but nevertheless continued to be practised more or less as folk medicine. Interest by Western doctors in acupuncture was quickened by President Nixon's visit to China in 1972. Since that time, medical interest in this subject has grown rapidly, being underpinned by a number of important medical discoveries as to why acupuncture may work.

The ancient Chinese considered that energy circulated in the body along specific channels, which they called meridians. This flow of energy has a direction. This is given on each meridian as flowing from point 1 to the point of the highest number on that meridian; for example, the bladder meridian runs from point 1 to 67 and the flow runs from 1 towards point 67. This is of great importance when using acupressure as the massage needs to be applied **in the direction of flow of the meridian**. All the charts in

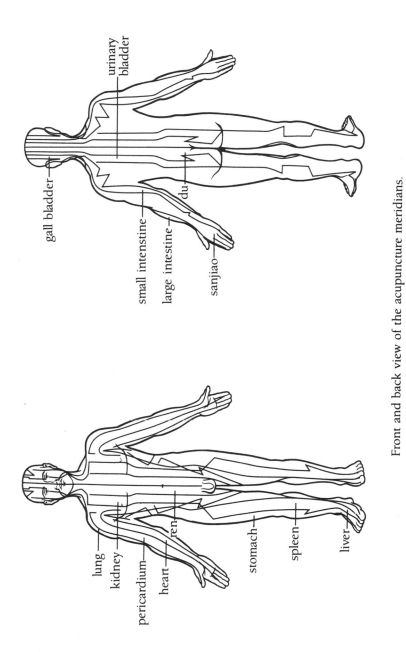

Front and back view of the acupuncture meridians.

this book have an arrow next to each point, showing the direction in which massage needs to be applied. Occasionally there are points in which the massage should be done in a circular (clockwise) fashion, but these points are not very common.

The ancient Chinese considered that the balance of energy from side to side, top to bottom and from the inside to the outside of the body was of great importance. They expressed this idea using their doctrine of Yin and Yang. Briefly, this considers that everything is an amalgam of opposites (the opposites being called Yin or Yang). Yang was associated with activity, fire, the sunny side of the hill or the male principle and Yin was associated with physical substance, water, the dark side of the hill or the female principle. The balance between these two opposites was considered to be constantly fluctuating – in other words, it was a dynamic balance. If a person was out of balance in an energetic sense then the principle of treatment would be to re-establish that balance. The Chinese therefore had an essentially vitalistic approach to the body and its physiology, in keeping with many ancient systems of medicine. It is interesting to reflect that modern Western medicine is the only system of medicine ever to have existed which does not have a vitalistic approach to health and disease.

The Chinese developed a highly complex and sophisticated system of empirical laws based on countless observations of illness and response to treatment, which resulted in a number of ground rules to guide a doctor as to how to improve his patient's condition. The astonishing fact is that application of these apparently odd-sounding laws appears to work in a highly significant proportion of patients. Clearly, if it did not do so then acupuncture would not have been adopted within both Western and Eastern cultures to such a degree.

The Chinese believed that as well as being in balance, the energy, or life force (which the Chinese called chi), had to be able to circulate freely around the meridians. If there is a break in its circulation anywhere then illness would result. For example, the traditional Chinese view of backache is that the chi circulating in the bladder meridian (which runs over the back, as shown in the following diagram) has got stuck somewhere. The way to remedy this is, in the simplest of possible terms, to insert a needle at the point of discomfort thus encouraging the flow to re-establish itself. Oddly enough, this relatively crude approach does work in a sufficient number of cases to raise more than passing interest.

Each meridian refers to a particular organ and the energy flow in that meridian should be taken as indicating the functional state of the organ. In other words, inserting a needle into a point on the liver meridian could be expected to affect liver function, the effect depending on the state of the patient at the time of treatment and on the actual point used.

A number of standard abbreviations are used in the treatment section and on the charts and are listed in the following table. There are twelve paired meridians, six running over the arms and onto the torso and six running up and down the legs and onto the trunk. There are two unpaired meridians, one running down the front mid-line and one down the back mid-line.

Abbreviations for the leg meridians:
G = Gall bladder
B = Urinary bladder
K = Kidney
Liv = Liver
S = Stomach
Sp = Spleen

The six paired arm meridians:
Li = Large intestine
Si = Small intestine
H = Heart
P = Pericardium
T = Triplewarmer
L = Lung

Unpaired mid-line meridians:
Cv = Conception vessel
Gv = Governor vessel

The use of acupressure allows you to stimulate points at which energy flow is blocked simply by applying deep massage to this point in the direction of flow of the channel.

Acupressure, whilst not being as effective as a needle, will work in many cases. **On no account, however, should you proceed to insert acupuncture needles into yourself. Leave this to a qualified practitioner.**

Ear Acupuncture
The Chinese discovered that in some cases pain anywhere on the

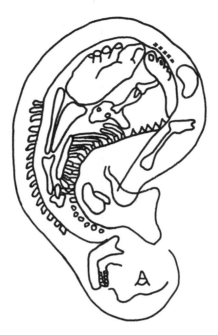

Representation of the body on the ear for the location of ear points.

body could be treated effectively and quickly by needling appropriate points on the outer ear. Recent research has shown that there appears to be a representation of the body on the outer ear, in an upside-down fashion (see diagram).

All you have to do is to locate where the problem is, find the equivalent site on the ear according to the diagram and treat the point. In some cases, relief is almost instantaneous. However, great accuracy in locating the point is required as the ear is small in relation to the body. One simple way, based on the observation that ear points for pain are sensitive to deep pressure, is to press with a blunt probe such as a matchstick or a sharp fingernail. On searching very carefully over the area on the ear where you think, according to the diagram, the correct energy point or points should be located, you should find one particular point which is more tender than surrounding points. Treat only those points which are sensitive to deep pressure. Use the ear which is on the same side as the problem; that is, the right ear for right-sided problems and the left ear for left-sided ones. If your problem is situated in the mid-line, such as in some cases of back pain, use the right ear if you are right-handed or the left ear if you are left-handed.

Ear acupressure is extremely effective, and really relies on searching carefully for a number of minutes in order to find the exact point. If the point is not tender then it is almost certainly not correct.

How Does it Work?
There are two currently favoured explanations as to the mode of action of acupuncture. One is the gate control theory of pain and the other is called the neuro-endocrine theory.

The gate control theory of pain
Nerves fibres are like large bundles of cables of various sizes, some thick and some thin. The thin fibres transmit the sensation of pain whilst the thick ones carry the sensation of touch. It has been found experimentally that if impulse transmission in the thick (touch) fibres can be increased, this selectively blocks conduction in the thin (pain) fibres by closing a gate consisting of specific nerve cells in the spinal cord. This therefore offers a useful means of controlling pain simply by using anything that increases transmission in the touch fibres. This is why deep pressure over an injured knee helps to relieve some of the pain. Acupuncture has been found to markedly increase transmission in the thick (touch) fibres. Acupressure achieves the same result, but it is important to apply deep pressure.

Neuro-endocrine theories
One of the most exciting recent discoveries in connection with acupuncture has been finding that needling of acupuncture points (energy points) causes the body to release its own natural pain killer, called endorphin. Endorphin is a protein molecule with very powerful pain-killing capabilities. It is released by many parts of the nervous system and is also related to the glandular or endocrine system, hence the term neuro-endocrine. It has been found that endorphin release is part of the explanation for some of the treatment successes following the use of acupressure.

Other theories
The most interesting explanations derive from the studies of very small electrical changes occurring at acupuncture points, which have been found to be capable of producing effects far in excess of

the tiny electrical change at the point responsible for triggering these effects. This is a new area of research and centres around looking at subtle electrical change over these energy points. It is now known that acupuncture points (energy points) are areas of low skin resistance, which means that these areas of skin conduct electricity into the body better than the surrounding skin, and a number of methods of applying electrical charge to acupuncture points have been developed. Another way of studying this is to make the points visible with the aid of sophisticated photographic technology. On doing this, the points appear like electrical pores on the skin.

Looking at these points side on – in other words, with the camera looking along the skin – shows another interesting feature in that a halo is present above the energy point. Preliminary studies show this halo to consist of charged particles called ions. In some cases, these are predominantly negative ions and in other cases predominantly positive ones.

THE TREATMENT OF SPECIFIC DISORDERS

This section is divided into the following parts:

1. Painful Disorders
2. Ear, Nose and Throat Problems
3. Heart and Circulatory Disorders
4. Abdominal Problems
5. Skin Disorders
6. Chest Diseases
7. Genito-urinary Problems
8. Miscellaneous Disorders
9. Sports Injuries.

You can either look up the section which you think will cover your disorder and use the points indicated, or find your condition by looking it up in the index.

This book makes no claims for curing the disorders mentioned, it merely points out simple ways in which these conditions may be helped. In some cases this will result in cure and in others it may bring some alleviation, but a proportion will not be helped at all. **It is essential to point out that a diagnosis of some sort is important, so if you do not know what is causing your pain, seek the opinion of a qualified doctor before you start treating yourself. Remember that pain is often a warning sign given by the body, so it must be heeded.** The majority of people with pain have it from a known cause such as a bad back or osteoarthritis. In these cases the pain has ceased to perform a useful alerting function and therefore needs treating in some way.

1. PAINFUL DISORDERS

Pain can be divided into acute (having been present for only a short time; that is, less than 2 weeks) and chronic (pain lasting longer than 2 weeks). Pain is perhaps the most common of all complaints. It occurs for many reasons and so a diagnosis of some sort is important. If you do know that your pain is coming from an arthritic joint then it is entirely reasonable to go ahead and treat it. If your pain is unexplained then your most urgent need is for a qualified medical opinion before you even think of treating it.

Sports Injuries, Sprains and Strains

These are common and often acutely painful conditions. It is always obvious what has caused them and therefore treatment can be applied immediately providing the possibility of any bone injury such as a fracture has been ruled out by appropriate x-ray investigation. Acupressure is an ideal method of self-treatment. Treating such injuries in the early stages is of considerable importance as it makes it far less likely that the condition will develop into a chronic painful problem. Sports injuries are dealt with specifically in Section 9.

Arthritis

This is perhaps the most common cause of chronic pain. There are two main sorts of arthritis: osteoarthritis, which in lay terms can be regarded as due to wear and tear; and rheumatoid arthritis which is a form of arthritis in which the joints have become inflamed. Osteoarthritic pain will respond better to acupressure than pain due to rheumatoid arthritis. This is not to say that rheumatoid arthritics will not derive benefit from it, but they are less likely to do so.

Back Pain

This is the most common reason for time lost from work. The pain is usually due to a narrowed intervertebral disc or discs in the lower part of the spine. Sometimes there is some associated osteoarthritis of the spine. Acupressure is an excellent way of treating this form of pain and should reduce the amount of time off work.

General Principles for the Use of Acupressure

1. Always treat the local tender points which the Chinese call Ah shi (literally translated, this means 'ouch' points). These can be

found by deep pressure over the painful area, noting those areas which are especially tender. Pressing hard enough to elicit some initial tenderness is of great importance, as this will lead to much more effective treatment.

2. In acute conditions (lasting less than 2 weeks) only a small number of treatments will be required - perhaps two or three.

3. In chronic conditions (lasting more than 2 weeks) many more treatments may be required - perhaps as many as twenty.

4. In acute conditions treatment can be as often as hourly.

5. In chronic conditions, treat 2 or 3 times weekly, increasing the interval between treatments as the condition improves.

6. If you can ask a friend or a relative to massage the relevant acupuncture points for you this will be more effective than massaging them yourself, especially if they are inaccessible such as on the back.

REMEMBER TO USE FIRM DEEP PRESSURE.

Headache (Migraine) Frontal

These points can be used for any headache occurring over the frontal (forehead) region of the head.

Migraine is a particular type of headache, often lasting many hours and accompanied by sensations of flashing lights, nausea and vomiting. It you have a migraine then treat using the points indicated as soon as any warning signs (such as flashing lights, etc.) appear even though the headache may not have started yet.

Treat each point for a number of minutes. During a migraine attack you can repeat treatment as often as every 3 to 4 hours. In all cases treat local tender points (Ah shi points). For the ear points search with a blunt object such as a matchstick or a fingernail so as to find the most tender point. Stimulate this vigorously with the finger nail or the tip of the matchstick.

Points:
B2, Yintang, G14, Li4, Liv3, S36 + ear point.

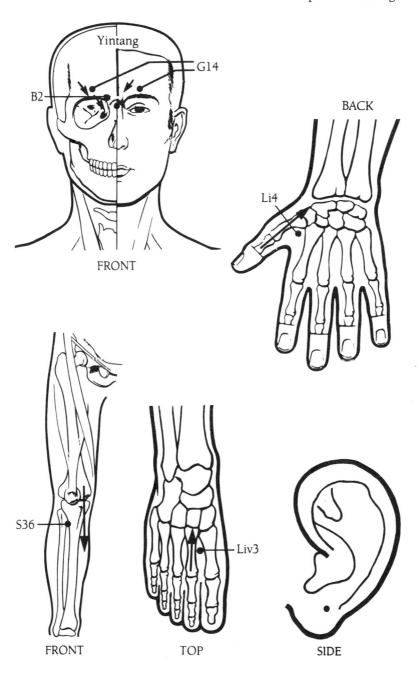

= direction of acupressure massage

Headache (Migraine) Occipital

This is a headache occurring over the back of the head. Many patients with occipital headaches have accompanying neck problems. It is well worth looking at the section on neck pain and also treating using those points. Always treat the local tender points.

Points:
G20, Gv15, B60, Li4, S36 + ear points.

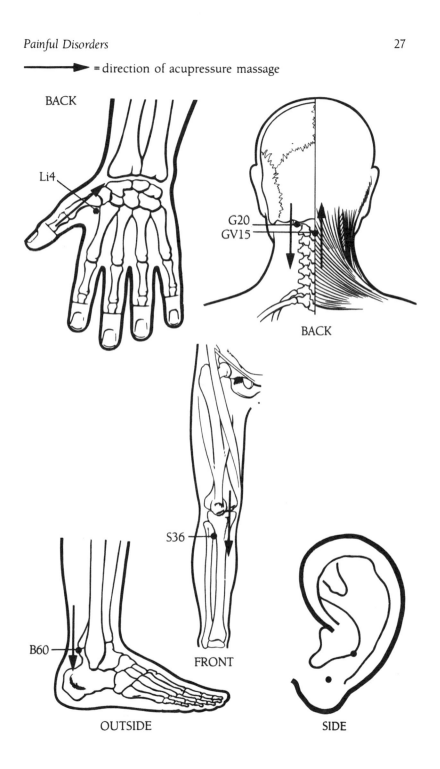

= direction of acupressure massage

BACK

Li4

G20
GV15

BACK

S36

FRONT

B60

OUTSIDE

SIDE

Headache (Migraine) Temporal

This is headache occurring on the side of the head. Always treat local tender points.

Points:
G20, Taiyang, G34, T5, S36 + ear point.

= direction of acupressure massage

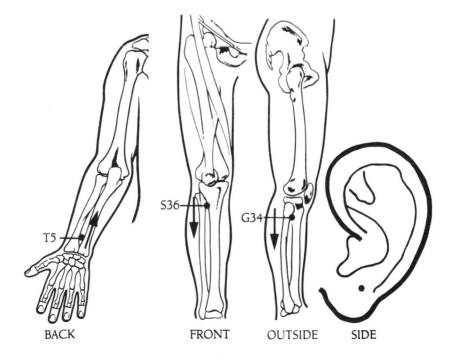

BACK

LEFT SIDE

BACK   FRONT   OUTSIDE   SIDE

Headache (Migraine) Vertex

This is a headache occurring on top of the head. Always treat local tender points.

Points:
Gv20, B60, Liv3, S36 + ear points.

= direction of acupressure massage

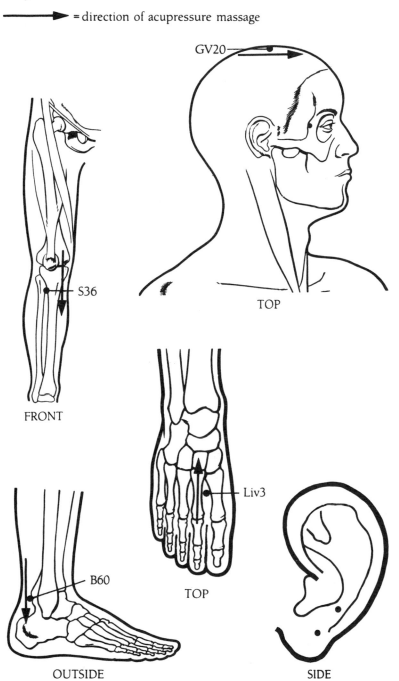

FRONT

S36

GV20

TOP

Liv3

TOP

B60

OUTSIDE

SIDE

Eye Pain

Eye pain can occur for many reasons but is perhaps most commonly associated with migraine where the patient often feels that the pain is behind the eyes. If eye pain is chronic then a qualified opthalmological opinion is mandatory.

Points:
Taiyang, Bl, Li4, Liv3 + ear point.

⟶ = direction of acupressure massage

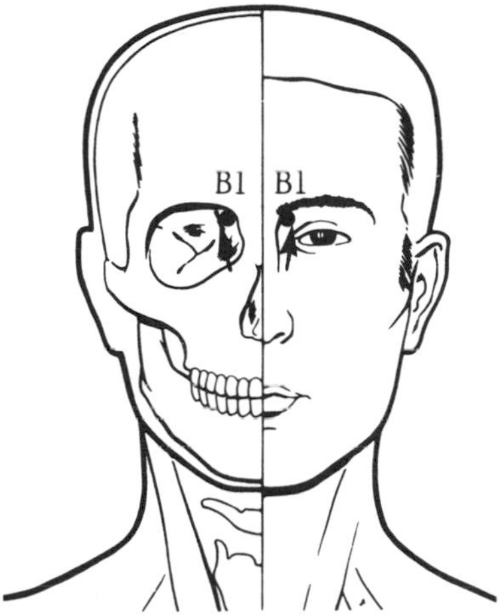

FRONT

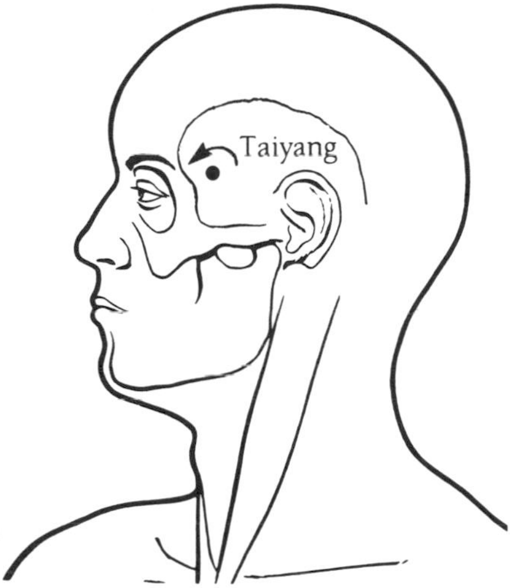

LEFT SIDE

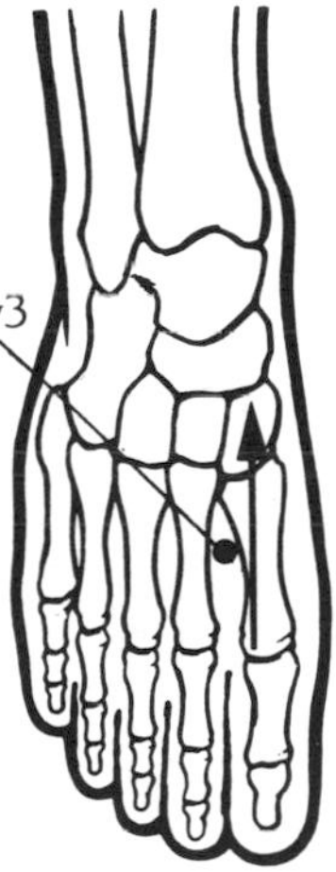

Taiyang

Bl Bl

BACK

Liv3

Li4

TOP

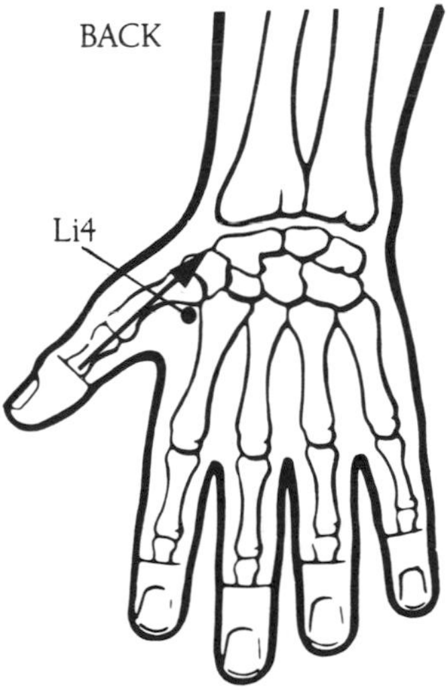

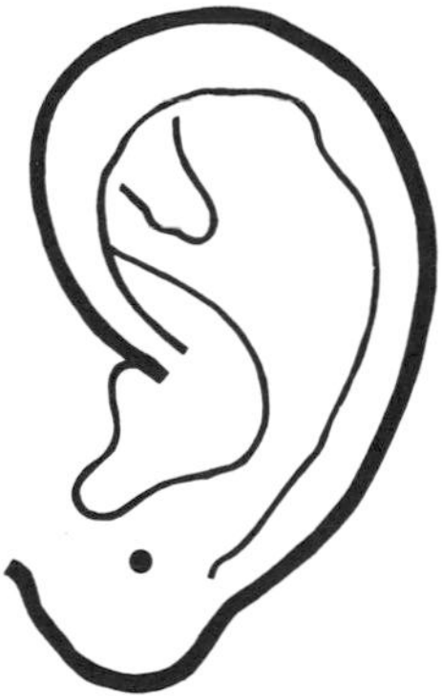

SIDE

Jaw Pain

This is sometimes accompanied by temporomandibular arthritis. Treatment with acupressure is often highly effective.

Points:
Li4, Si19, S7 + ear point.

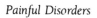 = direction of acupressure massage

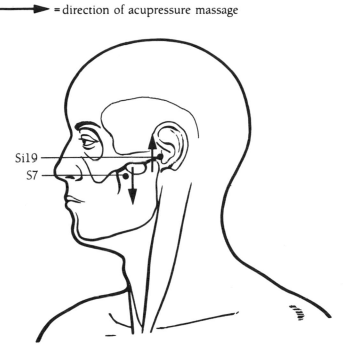

Si19
S7

LEFT SIDE

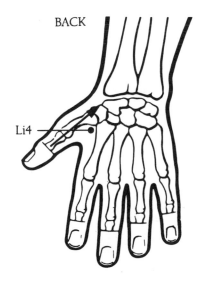

BACK

Li4

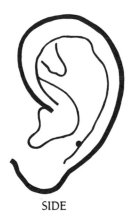

SIDE

Toothache (Lower Jaw)

The use of acupressure for the treatment of toothache should be regarded as a stop-gap prior to seeing the dentist, it is no substitute for proper dental attention.

Points:
Li4 + ear point.

Toothache (Upper Jaw)

The same comments apply as to toothache in the lower jaw.

Points:
S44 + ear point.

= direction of acupressure massage

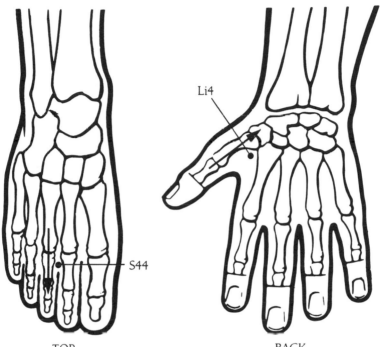

TOP

BACK

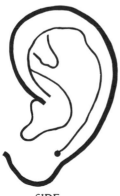

SIDE

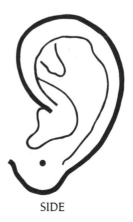

SIDE

Neck Pain

Neck pain is most commonly due to arthritis in the neck, sometimes called cervical spondylosis. A qualified osteopathic or chiropractic opinion is often helpful in the treatment of this problem although acupressure can be a highly effective method of treatment. Deep massage for a number of minutes is required on each of these points. It is quite hard work to treat neck pain effectively using acupressure. The treatment is best carried out by a relative or a friend, rather than attempting it yourself.

Points:
G21, Gv14, G20, Si3, Li4 + ear point.

= direction of acupressure massage

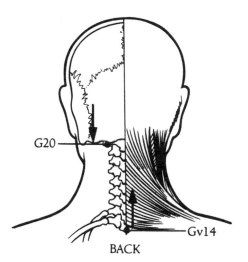

G20

Gv14

BACK

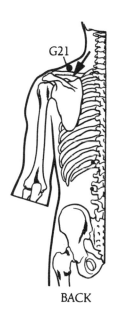

G21

BACK

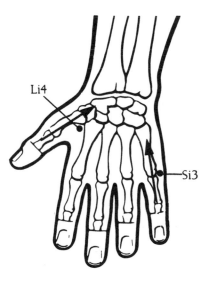

Li4

Si3

BACK

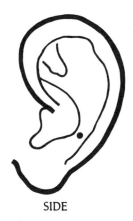

SIDE

Shoulder Pain

This is a common problem and should be treated vigorously. If shoulder pain is left for more than a month then a frozen shoulder may ensue in which stiffness of the joint as well as pain is a troublesome feature. In a chronically painful shoulder, which is also stiff, then physiotherapy is an essential approach to treatment, but, as in treating neck pain, vigorous and continuous massage lasting several minutes is needed for each point, together with all the local tender points (Ah Shi points).

Points:
Li15, T14, Li11, G21, S38, B57 + ear point.

= direction of acupressure massage

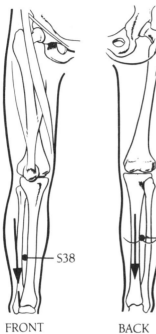

FRONT   BACK

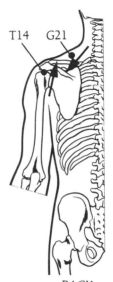

BACK

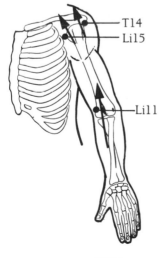

SIDE

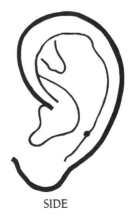

SIDE

Wrist Pain

This is most often due to strain caused by excessive use, but can occasionally be due to arthritis and is most commonly found in these situations in rheumatoid arthritis. Some patients have a condition called carpal tunnel syndrome which is due to compression of the median nerve as it passes deep to the front surface of the wrist. When this is compressed it gives rise to painful tingling sensations in the thumb, index, middle and part of the ring finger. Acupressure is an effective way of treating this and the most important point to use is P7.

Points:
Li5, Si5, T4, P7 + ear point.

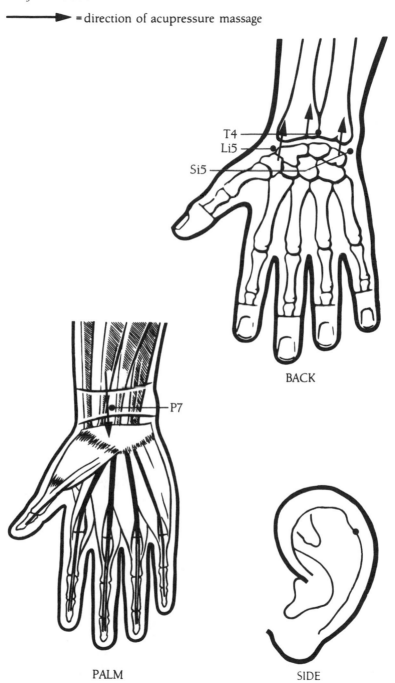

→ = direction of acupressure massage

T4
Li5
Si5

BACK

P7

PALM

SIDE

Hand Pain

This is most commonly due to injury when it is acute or in the chronic situation due to rheumatoid arthritis.

Points:
Li4 + extra points + ear point.

= direction of acupressure massage

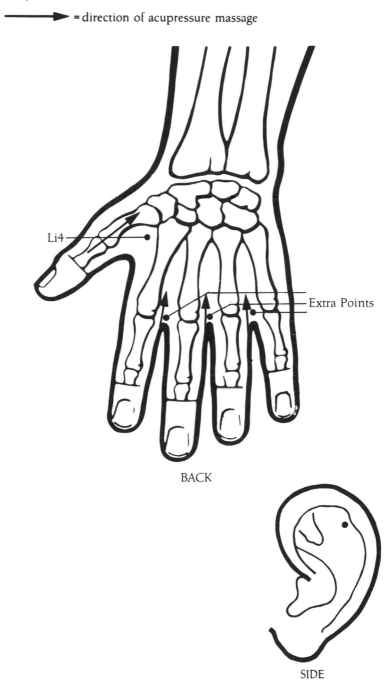

BACK

SIDE

Intercostal Neuralgia

This is due to irritation of the intercostal nerves which pass from the back at either side of the chest spine and run round just below each rib. They can cause pain and difficulty in breathing, but it is very important to diagnose accurately because its differential diagnosis if it occurs on the left side could be angina (heart pain) or if it occurs on either side could possibly be pleurisy. The treatment for angina and pleurisy involves other important measures and therefore acupressure on its own isn't the most appropriate form of treatment for either of these two conditions.

Points:

G34, Liv3, + local tender points and the other points as shown in the diagram depending on the site of neuralgia, + ear point.

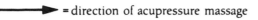 = direction of acupressure massage

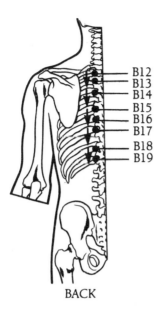

B12
B13
B14
B15
B16
B17
B18
B19

BACK

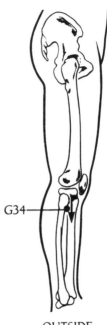

G34

OUTSIDE

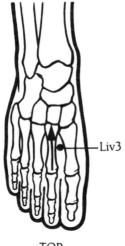

Liv3

TOP

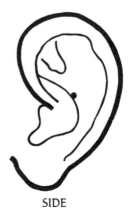

SIDE

Back Pain

This is most commonly due to narrowed discs in the lower lumbar spine. Occasionally it can be due to a so-called prolapsed intervertebral disc and in these cases the pain often extends down into the leg. If this does not respond satisfactorily to treatment then a competent osteopathic, chiropractic or orthopaedic opinion should be sought. A very small proportion of these cases will require surgery and removal of the protruding disc. In all cases, however, it is essential to try conservative measures first. Acupressure is well worth a try in these cases and is often successful at relieving much chronic low back pain. Firm pressure for 1 minute on each point is essential if the treatment is to be successful.

Points:
B31, B25, B40, G30 + local tender points as is standard for all painful conditions + ear point.

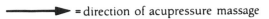

= direction of acupressure massage

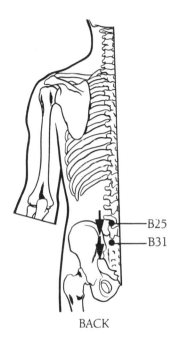

B25
B31

BACK

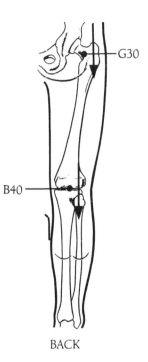

G30

B40

BACK

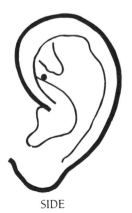

SIDE

Hip Pain

This is most commonly due to arthritis in the hip. If treatment is unsuccessful then a competent orthopaedic opinion should be sought. Firm pressure for some minutes over each point is essential.

Points:
Local tender points, G29, S31, G30, G34 + ear point.

= direction of acupressure massage

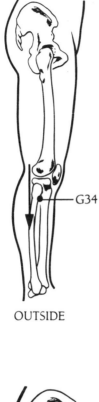

OUTSIDE

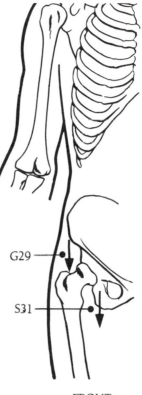

FRONT

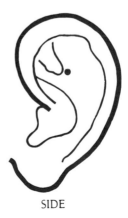

SIDE

SIDE

Knee Pain

This is most commonly due to arthritis of the knee in older people, and in younger people it can be due to damage to the cartilages present in the knee joint. Occasionally these cartilages are torn due to a twisting injury as sometimes occurs in football. If the knee locks as a result of the torn cartilage getting stuck in the centre of the joint then removal of the cartilage is usually required. As a general rule the use of acupressure is highly effective in treating knee pain. Deep, firm pressure is essential.

Points:
Xiyan (the so-called eyes of the knees), Sp9, B40 + ear point.

——————► = direction of acupressure massage

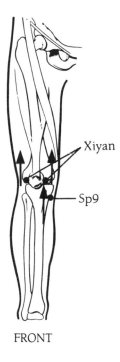

Xiyan

Sp9

FRONT

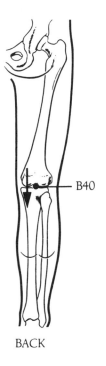

B40

BACK

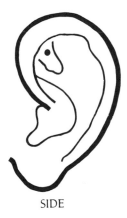

SIDE

Ankle Pain

This is most commonly due to arthritis of the ankle when chronic and to sprain when acute.

Points:
S41, G40, Sp5 + ear point.

➤ = direction of acupressure massage

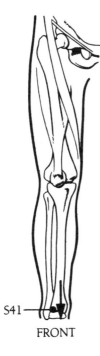

S41—

FRONT

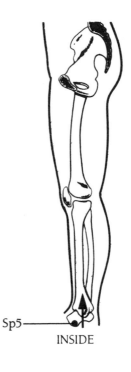

Sp5—

INSIDE

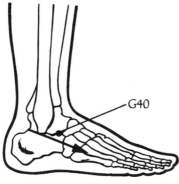

G40

OUTSIDE

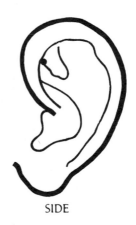

SIDE

Foot Pain

This can be due to strain, as in the case of joggers who have perhaps been over-enthusiastic, or can be due to arthritis, most commonly rheumatoid arthritis.

Points:
Extra points + local tender points + ear point.

→ = direction of acupressure massage

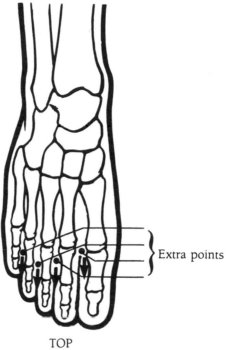

} Extra points

TOP

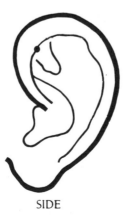

SIDE

Sciatica

This is pain radiated down the sciatic nerve which runs down the back of the leg onto the outer aspect of the foot. Sciatica does not always mean that there is a prolapsed intervertebral disc present. The majority of cases of sciatica respond well to a conservative approach using vigorous acupressure. A very small proportion will require surgery.

Points:
B31, 32, 33, 37, 40, G30 + local tender points + ear points.

➡️ = direction of acupressure massage

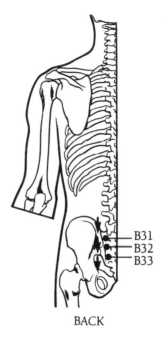

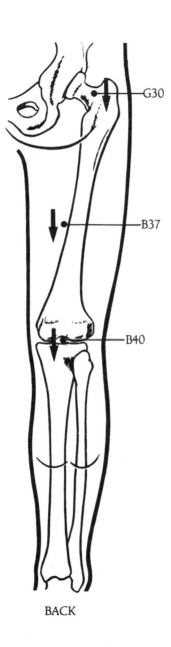

BACK

BACK

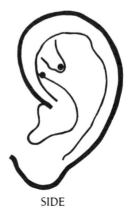

SIDE

Cramp

This is due to spasm in the blood vessels supplying the muscles of the leg, particularly the calf. Treatment need not be given when the cramp is actually occurring since treatment outside this time should reduce the incidence of cramp and eventually stop it occurring altogether.

Points:
P6, B57, B40 + ear points.

——————▶ =direction of acupressure massage

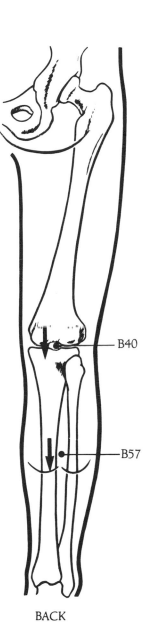

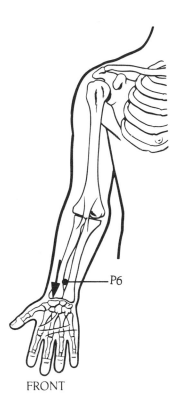

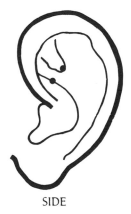

B40

B57

FRONT

P6

BACK

SIDE

Shingles

This is an infection due to the herpes zoster virus (which is the same as the chicken pox virus). It results in a vesicular rash, often present in a diagonal orientation running downwards from the back towards the front. It is often situated somewhere over the chest or the abdomen. It is a particularly painful condition and should be treated vigorously. Acupressure can be regarded as an effective method of treatment. In some cases the pain from shingles can become chronic, giving rise to a condition known as post-herpetic neuralgia. This is much more difficult to treat but acupressure is certainly worth a try. It is all the more essential that shingles is treated vigorously in the acute stage, as indicated here. Treat a number of points around the rash. This will involve many points if the rash is extensive, perhaps as many as twenty or thirty. Most of these points will be tender. Do not treat points in or on the rash itself. Also use Liver 3. Search for ear points, choosing them according to the area affected as shown on the diagram of the body on the ear on page 15. Treatment can be twice daily in the acute situation.

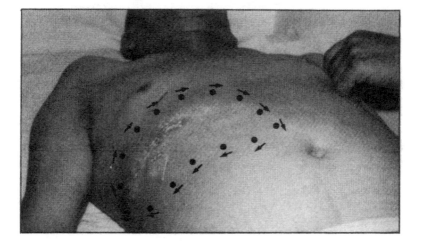 = direction of acupressure massage

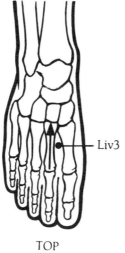

Liv3

TOP

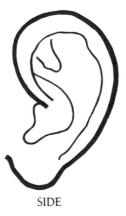

SIDE

Dysmenorrhoea (Painful Periods)

This is a common problem and acupressure is often an effective method of treating it. Other measures may also be necessary. One of the useful approaches which can be applied at home is to take zinc supplements and Vitamin B6.

Points:
S36, Sp6, Cv6, B31, Liv3 + ear points.

= direction of acupressure massage

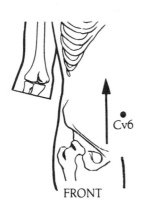

Cv6

FRONT

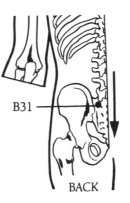

B31

BACK

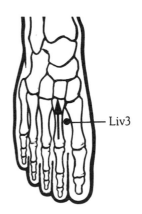

Liv3

TOP

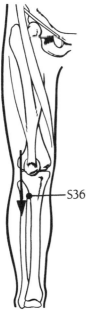

S36

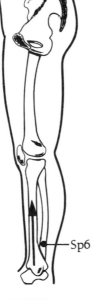

Sp6

FRONT

INSIDE

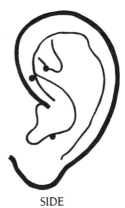

SIDE

Renal (Kidney) Colic

This is pain due to the passage of a hard object down the ureter, which is the tube passing from the kidney to the bladder. This is usually due to a kidney stone. The pain is often very severe and the patient characteristically rolls around on the floor.

Acupressure is often a useful method of treatment. The ear point is particularly important for this condition.

Points:

K3, B20 + local tender points + the ear point. In renal colic the use of the ear point is very important.

——————▶ = direction of acupressure massage

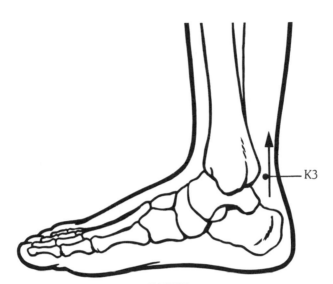

INSIDE

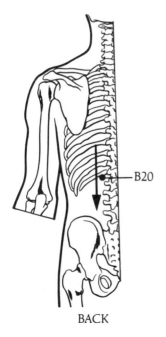

BACK

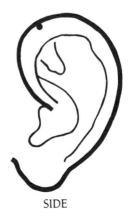

SIDE

2. EAR, NOSE AND THROAT PROBLEMS

Laryngitis

Laryngitis is nearly always an acute problem which involves loss of voice. It is most often due to a viral infection. Chronic laryngitis should always lead the sufferer to seek a qualified E.N.T. opinion to rule out any more serious problems.

Points:
Li4, L7, Cv22 + ear point.

= direction of acupressure massage

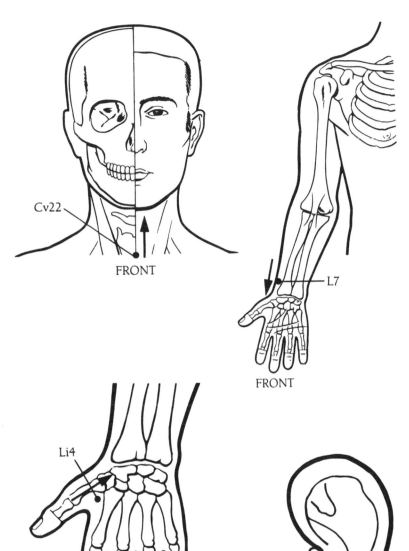

Cv22

FRONT

L7

FRONT

Li4

BACK

SIDE

Sinusitis

Sinusitis is very common indeed and can occur either in the maxillary sinuses which lie deep in the face below the eyes on both sides, or the frontal sinuses which lie above the eyes on either side of the bridge of the nose. People with sinusitis should consider other methods as well as using acupressure in order to help their problem. Additional approaches centre around diet, and the avoidance of foods which produce excessive mucous such as milk and dairy products and red meat should be considered. Attention should be paid to bowel function. Even slight constipation in those people predisposed to sinusitis can lead to troublesome chronic problems in this area. The reason that the colon is connected to the sinuses is that the large intestine meridian ends on the sinuses and has a connection with the large intestine itself (ie. the colon).

Points:
Li20, Li4, Sp6, Yintang + ear point.

➤ = direction of acupressure massage

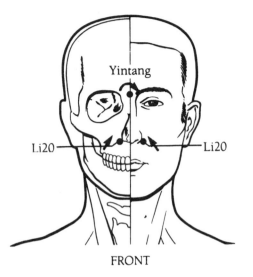

Yintang

Li20   Li20

FRONT

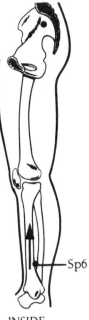

Sp6

INSIDE

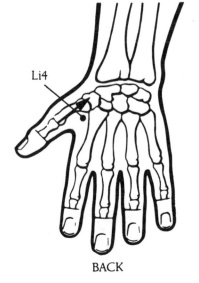

Li4

BACK

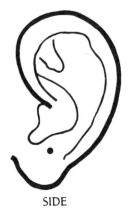

SIDE

Mouth Ulcers

Mouth ulcers are particularly common and troublesome complaints. They are often very painful.

Points:
Li4, S36 + ear point.

⟶ = direction of acupressure massage

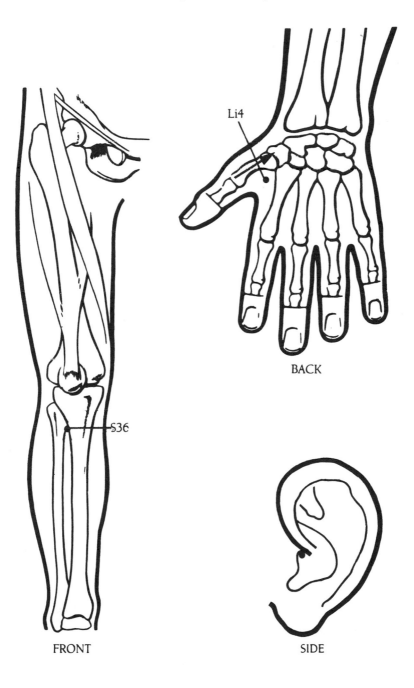

FRONT

BACK

SIDE

Nose Bleeds (Epistaxis)

Recurrent nose bleeding is common in children and acupressure offers a method of reducing the time of the nose bleed and so minimizing blood loss.

Points:
G20, P6, Li4 + ear point.

= direction of acupressure massage

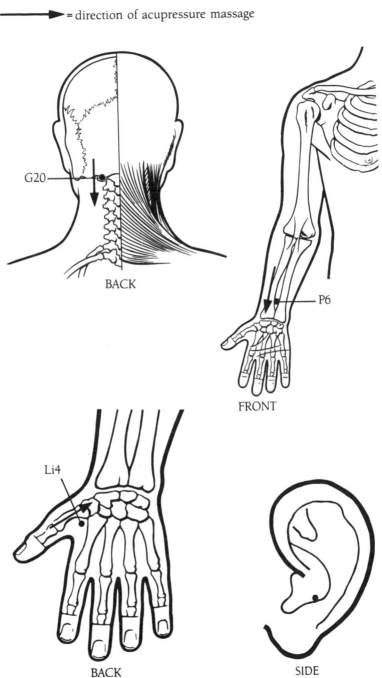

Tinnitus (Ringing in the Ears)

Tinnitus is often perceived as a high-pitched whistling sound which is much more noticeable in quiet surroundings. It often goes along with degeneration of the hearing nerve; in other words, it is often accompanied by hearing loss. It is a very difficult condition indeed to treat, but acupressure offers relief in approximately half of patients with tinnitus. This represents a considerable improvement on conventional approaches to this problem.

Points:
K3, Si3, T17, Si19, G20 + ear points.

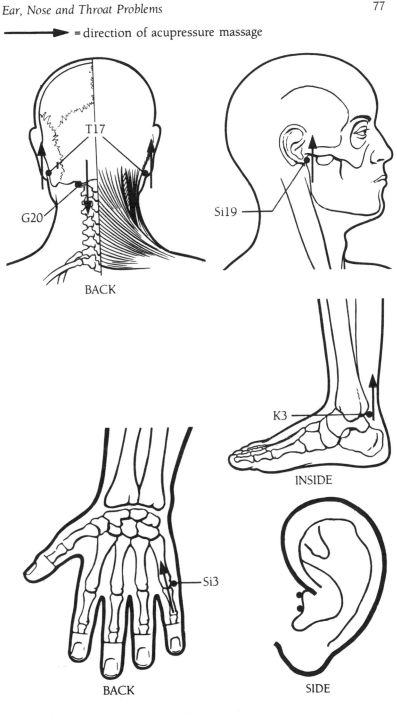

= direction of acupressure massage

Tonsillitis

Tonsillitis, or sore throat, is most often due to a viral infection. In some cases it can be due to a bacterial infection, so if no improvement follows from the approach suggested then a doctor ought to be consulted and almost certainly a course of antibiotics will be given.

Points:
Li4, S36 + ear point.

= direction of acupressure massage

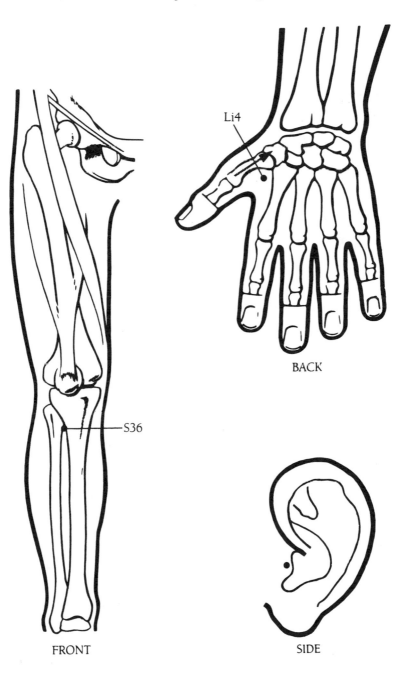

FRONT

BACK

SIDE

3. HEART AND CIRCULATORY DISORDERS

Angina

Angina is pain occurring on the left side of the chest, radiating down the left arm and occasionally up into the left side of the jaw. It is due to a lack of blood supply to the heart muscle. Often other measures are required: for example, a change in diet avoiding fatty foods such as red meats, milk and dairy products; stopping smoking; and attention to lifestyle to remove stress and excessive physical activity. **Acupressure can only be regarded as a symptomatic approach to this problem.**

Points:
Cv17, P6, H7 + ear point on the left side only.

⟶ = direction of acupressure massage

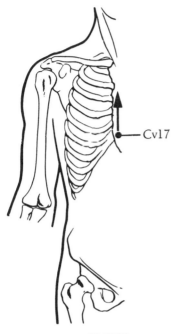

Cv17

FRONT

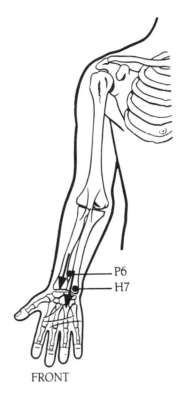

P6
H7

FRONT

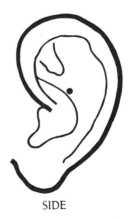

SIDE

Chilblains

These are relatively common in cold climates and acupressure offers a useful method of treatment.

Points:
P6, S36 + local points around the chilblains + ear point.

→ = direction of acupressure massage

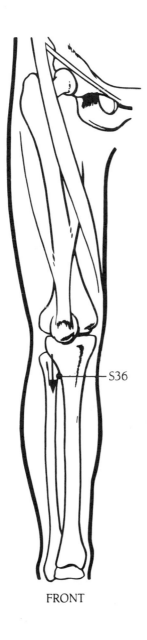

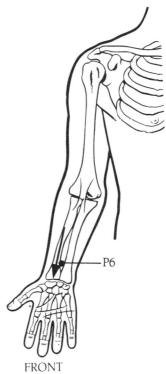

P6

FRONT

S36

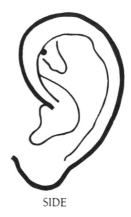

FRONT

SIDE

84

High Blood Pressure (Hypertension)

Hypertension is common in the civilized world. Effective treatment of hypertension is essential as otherwise the patient runs the risk of having a stroke. It is therefore essential that treatment is monitored by either taking the blood pressure yourself or getting a doctor to take it for you. If acupressure doesn't work then you will have to fall back on to conventional anti-hypertensive drugs.

Points:
P6, K3, S36 + ear point.

= direction of acupressure massage

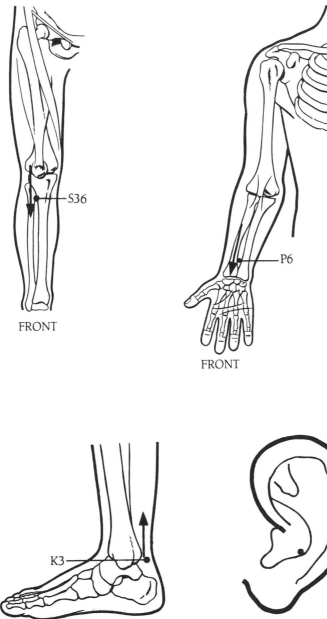

FRONT

S36

FRONT

P6

INSIDE

K3

SIDE

Palpitations

Palpitations are due to the heart beating irregularly. It often feels like a fluttering in the left side of the chest. It is rarely serious, but it is worth considering other methods as well as using acupressure in order to control it. In some cases palpitations are caused by reactions to foods, particularly coffee. Patients with palpitations would therefore be well advised to avoid coffee altogether. This alone can produce a great improvement. Acupressure can also help.

Points:
P6, H7 + ear points.

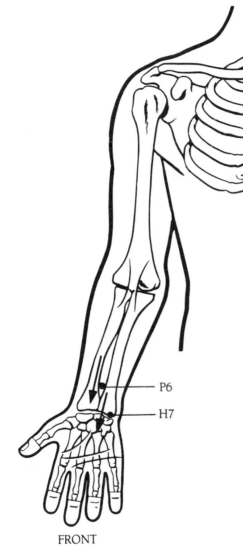

= direction of acupressure massage

P6

H7

FRONT

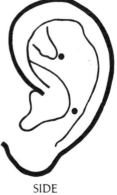

SIDE

4. ABDOMINAL PROBLEMS

Abdominal Distension

Recurrent abdominal distension is a common problem, particularly in women. It is most commonly due to dysfunction in the colon. Some cases can be helped enormously by acupressure but often a dietary approach has to be considered as well. The most effective approach is to avoid mucous-producing foods such as milk and dairy products, red meat and eggs.

Points:
S36, Sp6, S25 + ear points.

➤ = direction of acupressure massage

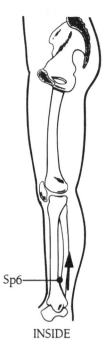

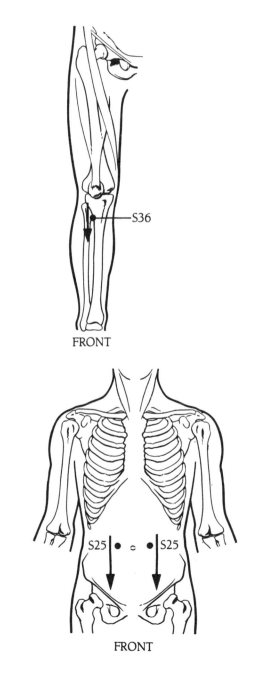

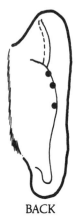

FRONT   INSIDE

FRONT   BACK

Colitis

Colitis is inflammation of the colon. The symptoms are often loose bowels, mucous and sometimes blood passed rectally. Conventional approaches to colitis can sometimes be alarming, involving steroids and in the worst possible cases removal of the affected part of the colon. Therefore simple approaches such as using acupressure are welcome alternatives. Attention to diet is also necessary as in some cases colitis can be due to food sensitivity. The most common foods involved are milk and dairy products, so it is well worth considering cutting these out of the diet.

Points:
S36, Sp6, S40 + ear points.

→ = direction of acupressure massage

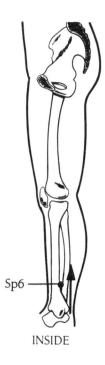

Sp6

INSIDE

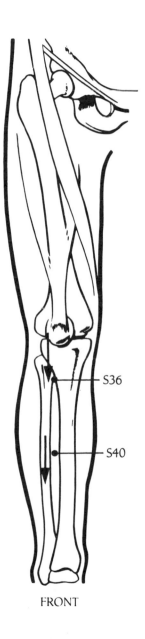

S36

S40

FRONT

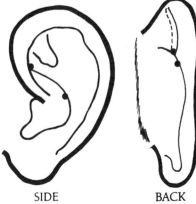

SIDE   BACK

Constipation

All people with constipation should pay attention to their diet and should go onto a high roughage diet eating wholemeal bread (never white bread), lots of vegetables, particularly raw carrots, cauliflower and cabbage, and avoiding processed foods as much as possible. It is also a good idea to eat plenty of fresh fruit.

Points:
Liv2, Li4, S25 + ear points.

⟶ = direction of acupressure massage

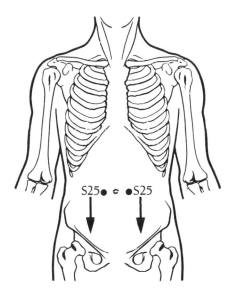

FRONT

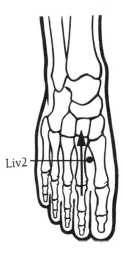

TOP

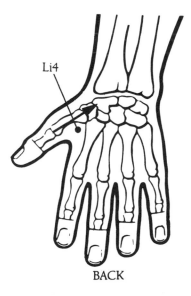

BACK

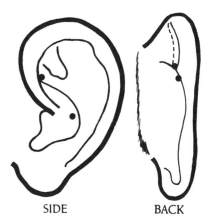

SIDE   BACK

Diarrhoea

Diarrhoea, if it is chronic, is commonly due to colitis. If acute it may be infective. Acute infective diarrhoea is most often due to a virus but can in some cases be due to a more serious infection such as salmonella. In these cases appropriate medical advice should be sought in order to stop the problem spreading to friends and relatives. If diarrhoea is accompanied by blood, medical advice should always be sought prior to treatment.

Points:
S36, Sp6, S25, Cv6 + ear points.

→ = direction of acupressure massage

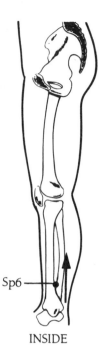

S36

Sp6

FRONT   INSIDE

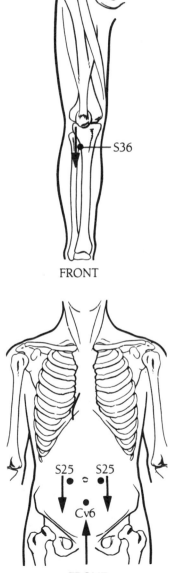

S25   S25

Cv6

FRONT

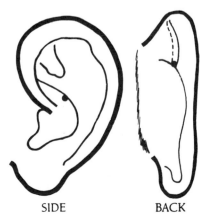

SIDE   BACK

Haemorrhoids

Haemorrhoids are varicosities of the veins around the lower end of the rectum. One of the points used by the Chinese is situated on the top of the head. The mind boggles as to how this could possibly help haemorrhoids, but I well remember seeing a case in China of prolapsed haemorrhoids reducing in front of my eyes at the same time as the point on the top of the head (Gv20) was stimulated. I can offer no explanation as to why this point should work.

Points
Gv20, Gv1, B40 + ear points.

──────▶ = direction of acupressure massage

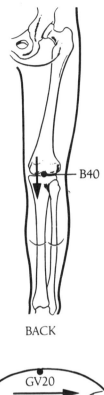

BACK

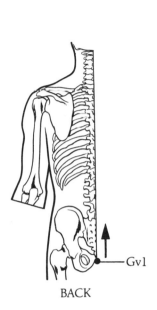

BACK

TOP   SIDE   BACK

Heartburn

Heartburn is due to regurgitation of stomach acid up the oesophagus. It is sometimes an accompaniment of hiatus hernia where the top part of the stomach (the so-called fundus) herniates up into the chest. This is often associated with patients who are overweight and therefore an attempt at weight loss can be very helpful.

Points:
Cv12, S36 + ear points.

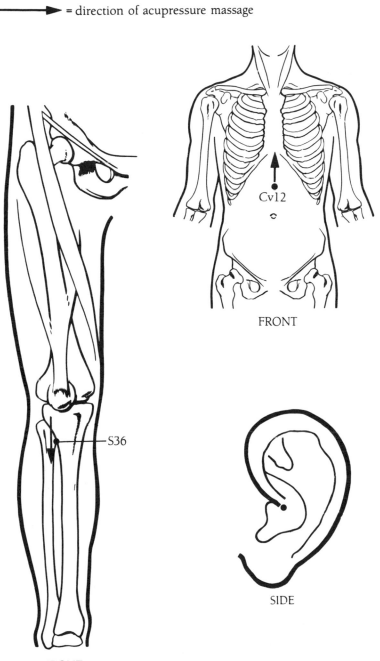

= direction of acupressure massage

Cv12

FRONT

S36

FRONT

SIDE

Liver Trouble

Liver trouble is often accompanied by general biliousness and intolerance of fatty foods. It is worth considering reducing fat intake as the liver copes with a good deal of the fat in the diet.

Points:
Liv3, Liv14, Cv12 + ear point.

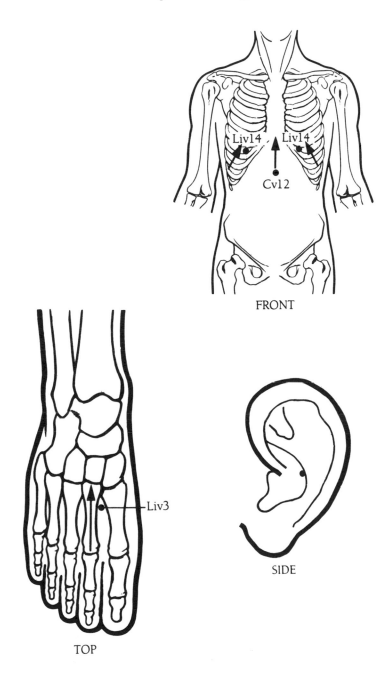

= direction of acupressure massage

Nausea

Nausea can occur for many, many reasons, but acupressure offers a useful approach.

Points:
P6, S36 + ear point.

= direction of acupressure massage

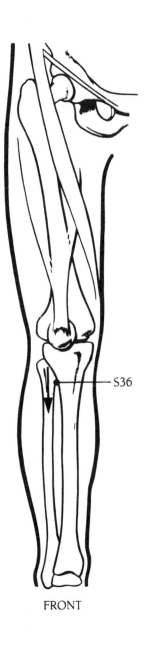

S36

FRONT

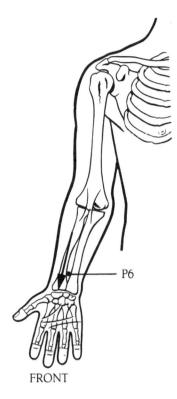

P6

FRONT

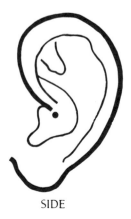

SIDE

Upper Abdominal Pain

Upper abdominal pain is very common indeed and a diagnosis of some sort is absolutely essential. Most commonly, the problem arises in the stomach – for example, due to a peptic ulcer – or is due to gall bladder problems.

Points:
T6, Sp6, Sp9, Liv14 + ear point.

= direction of acupressure massage

BACK

Liv14

FRONT

T6

Sp9

Sp6

INSIDE   SIDE   BACK

5. SKIN DISORDERS

Acne

Acne is common in teenagers and many topically applied creams are recommended. Unfortunately the results from these creams are generally disappointing. It is worthwhile considering other approaches as well as acupressure, amongst which attention to bowel function is top of the list. A change of diet to a high roughage, low mucous diet (wholemeal bread, lots of raw vegetables and avoidance of red meat, milk and dairy products, eggs and particularly chocolate) will help here.

Points:
Li4, S7, S36 + ear points.

→ = direction of acupressure massage

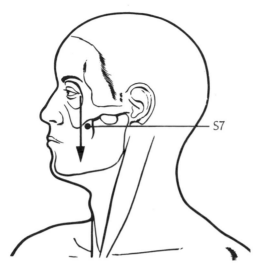

LEFT SIDE

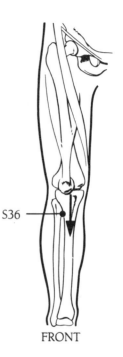

FRONT

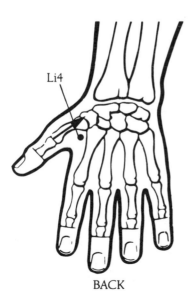

BACK

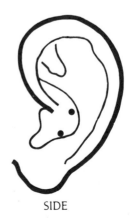

SIDE

Eczema

Eczema is an allergic inflammation of the skin. It commonly occurs in skin folds such as the elbows and knees. Conventional approaches to eczema centre around the use of steroid creams. These are often problematical as long-term use causes skin thinning. Therefore any alternative approach which isn't harmful is very welcome. Eczema can in some cases be due to food sensitivity. The most common foods implicated are milk and dairy products, and eggs. Experimenting in avoidance of these foods can be useful.

Points:
Liv3, S36 + ear points.

⟶ = direction of acupressure massage

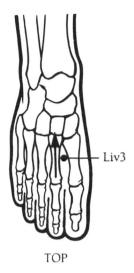

TOP

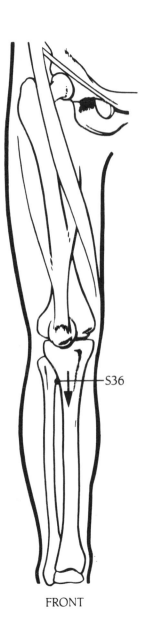

FRONT

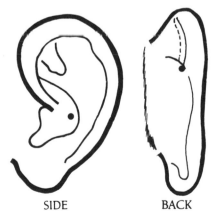

SIDE   BACK

6. CHEST DISEASES

Asthma

Acupressure can offer a useful approach to asthma but it should not be taken as a complete substitue for drugs which are usually taken as inhalers to dilate the bronchial tubes. This particularly applies in severe attacks when if no result is obtained with acupressure then bronchodilator drugs should be resorted to.

Points:
Cv17, B13, S36, K7 + ear point.

➤ = direction of acupressure massage

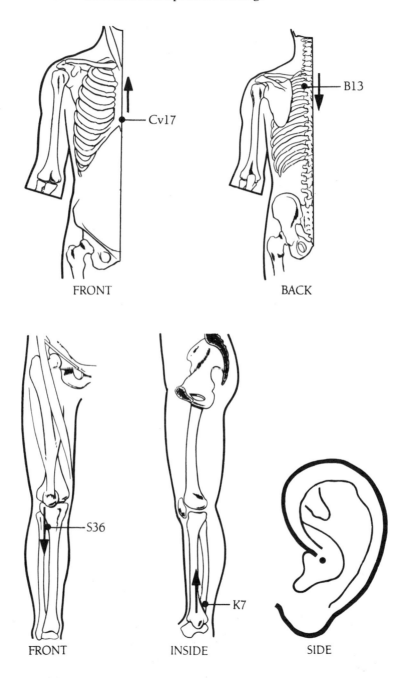

FRONT   BACK

FRONT   INSIDE   SIDE

Bronchitis

Bronchitis can occur just during the winter months or can be present all the year round. People with bronchitis produce copious amounts of sticky phlegm which they cough up off the chest. It is important that patients with bronchitis should stop smoking and avoid situations with air pollution such as enclosed garages, etc.

Points:
S40, Sp6, B13, Cv17 + ear point.

→ = direction of acupressure massage

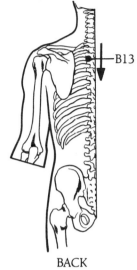

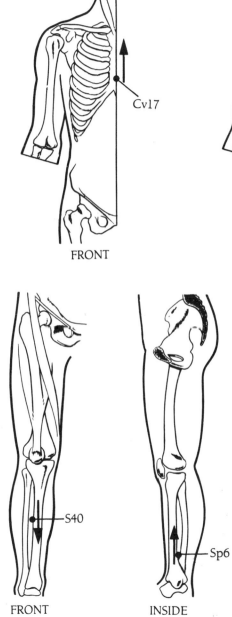

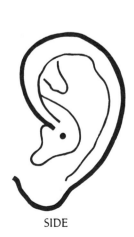

7. GENITO-URINARY PROBLEMS

Bed-wetting (Enuresis)

Acupressure offers a useful approach to enuresis and is particularly worth trying in children.

Points:
K3, Sp6, Cv4 + ear points.

━━━━▶ = direction of acupressure massage

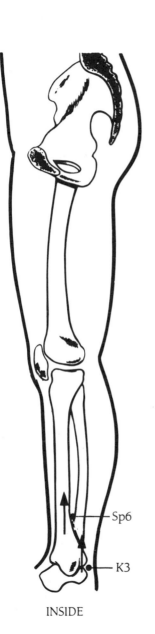

INSIDE

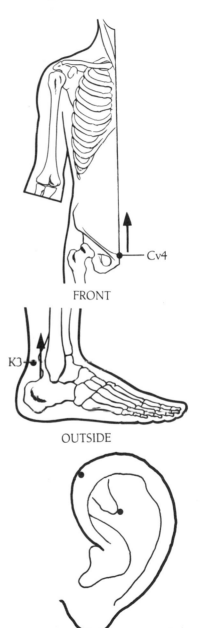

FRONT

OUTSIDE

SIDE

Incontinence (Urinary)

This is involuntary release of urine. It is common in older people, particularly men with enlarged prostate glands (situated around the base of the bladder). In some cases acupressure can alleviate this problem.

Points:
Cv2, SP6 + ear point.

→ = direction of acupressure massage

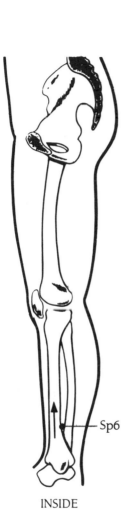

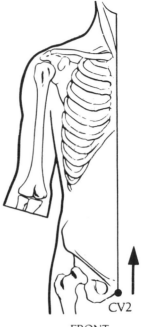

CV2

FRONT

Sp6

INSIDE

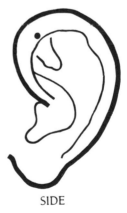

SIDE

Urinary Retention

This occurs most often in elderly men and is most commonly due to enlargement of the prostate gland situated at the base of the bladder. If it is recurrent then it is important that the opinion of a urological surgeon is sought. The approach with acupressure can be very useful if the retention is caught early.

Points:
Sp6, Sp9, B28 + ear point.

→ = direction of acupressure massage

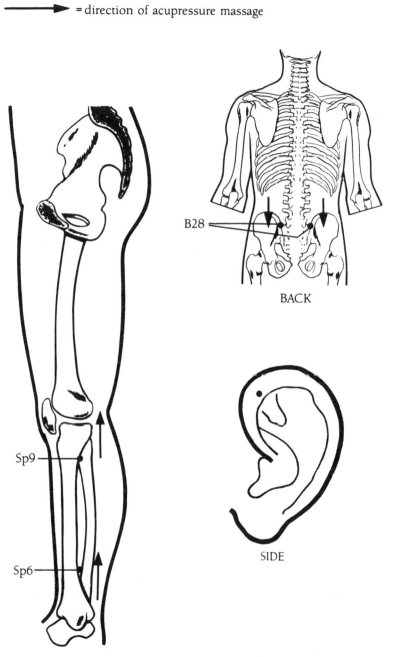

B28

BACK

Sp9

Sp6

INSIDE

SIDE

8. MISCELLANEOUS DISORDERS

Conjunctivitis

Conjunctivitis is inflammation of the outer coating of the eyeball. If conjunctivitis is recurrent then an opthalmological opinion should be sought.

Points:
Liv3, S36, Taiyang + ear point.

→ = direction of acupressure massage

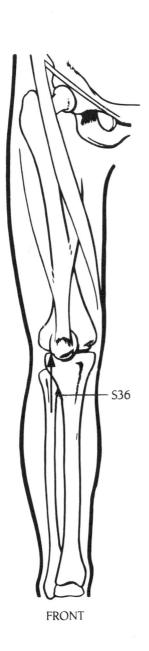

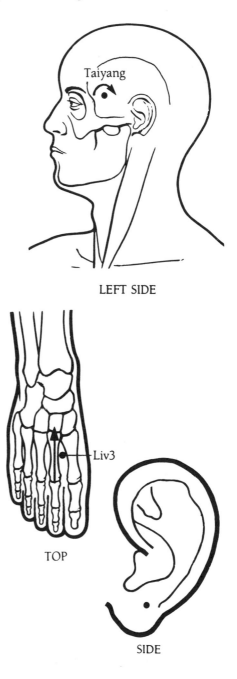

FRONT

S36

Taiyang

LEFT SIDE

Liv3

TOP

SIDE

Decreased Libido

Acupressure can be a useful approach to decreased libido and will work in a small proportion of cases. **This treatment cannot be regarded as an aphrodisiac.**

Points:
Sp6, S36, Cv6 + ear point.

➤ = direction of acupressure massage

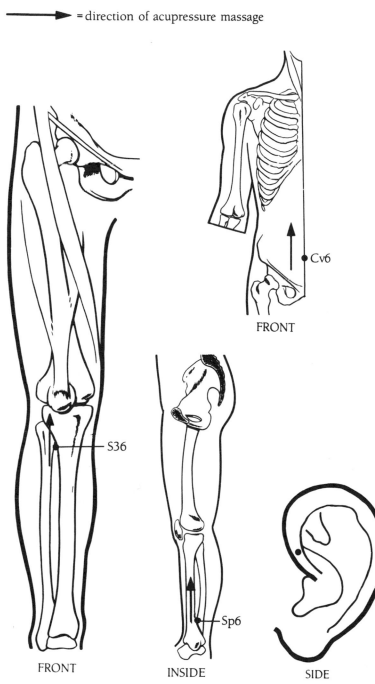

FRONT

S36

Cv6

FRONT

Sp6

FRONT   INSIDE   SIDE

Fever

Acupressure offers a symptomatic approach to fever but the cause must also be treated. This may involve a course of antibiotics if a bacterial infection is present.

Points:
Gv14, LiII, Li4 + ear point.

⟶ = direction of acupressure massage

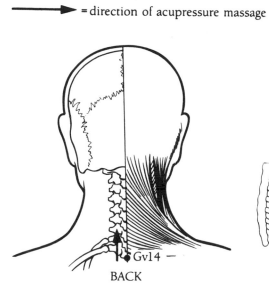

Gvl4 —

BACK

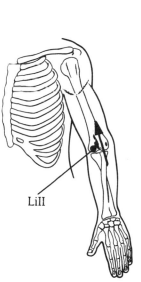

LiI1

SIDE

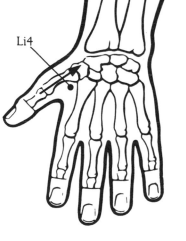

Li4

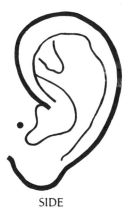

SIDE

Excessive Sweating

Sweating can occur for many reasons such as fever, general debilitation, stress and tension. In some cases acupressure can be a useful treatment approach.

Points:
H6, K7 + ear point.

= direction of acupressure massage

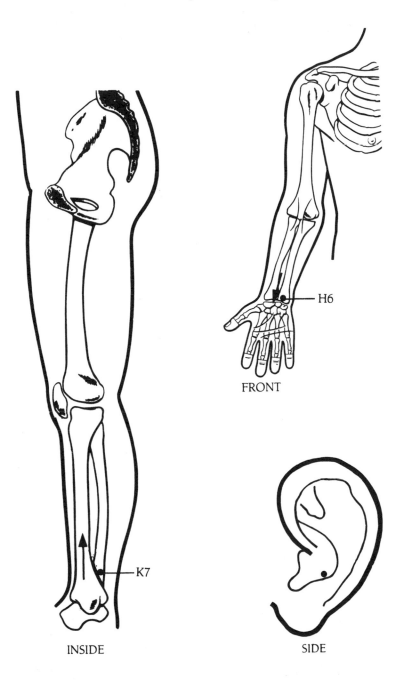

H6

FRONT

K7

INSIDE

SIDE

Fainting Attacks

If fainting attacks occur regularly then a medical opinion should be sought. If no satisfactory treatment is offered then it is perfectly reasonable to try acupressure as detailed here.

Points:
Cv26, H7, P6 + ear points.

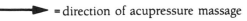 = direction of acupressure massage

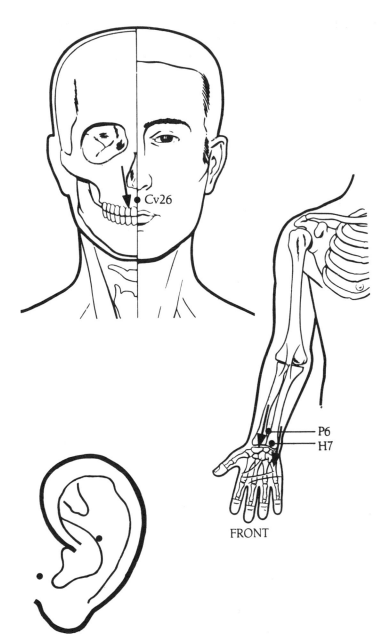

Cv26

P6
H7

FRONT

SIDE

Hiccoughs

Hiccoughs can be a particularly troublesome complaint. Acupressure offers a useful approach. It is often worth combining this with drinking a glass of cold water whilst holding the nose and therefore holding the breath. This has the effect of splinting the diaphragm as hiccoughs are a spasmodic contraction of the diaphragm.

Points:
B17, S36 + ear point.

━━━━━━▶ = direction of acupressure massage

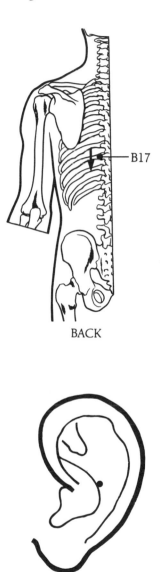

B17

BACK

SIDE

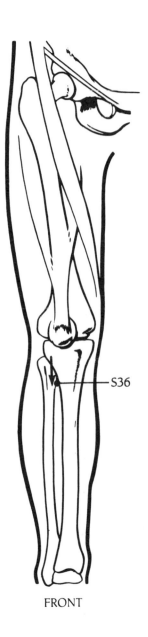

S36

FRONT

Hay Fever

Hay fever is an allergic reaction to grass and flower pollens and is therefore a seasonal affliction. A homoeopathic approach using homoeopathic grass and flower pollens is well worth considering. Acupressure can be a useful adjunct and will sometimes work on its own.

Points:
Liv3, S36 + ear point.

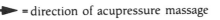 = direction of acupressure massage

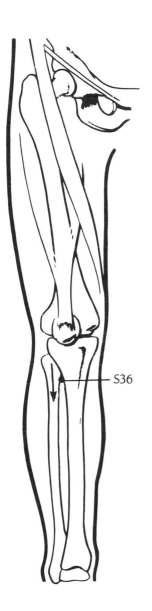

S36

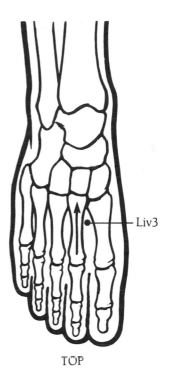

Liv3

TOP

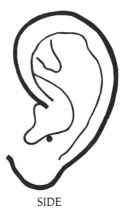

SIDE

Hot Flushes

Hot flushes most often occur at the time of the menopause. They are due to a hormonal imbalance which occurs at this time. They are particularly troublesome to treat and acupressure offers a safe and often effective method of coping with them. Treatment should be carried out on a regular basis even though no hot flushes may be occurring at the time of treatment.

Points:
S36, Sp6 + ear points.

➤ = direction of acupressure massage

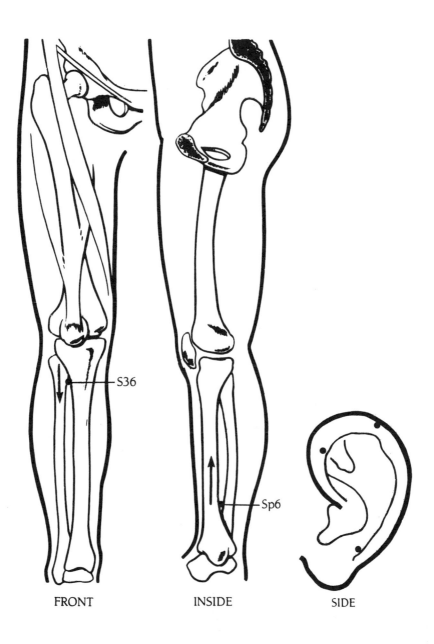

FRONT   INSIDE   SIDE

Insomnia

This is lack of sleep, which most commonly occurs for no apparent reason, therefore purely symptomatic approaches (sleeping tablets) are the rule. Acupressure can help to reduce the dependence of the patient on sleep-inducing drugs.

Points:
H7, Sp6, K3 + ear point.

⟶ = direction of acupressure massage

K3

INSIDE

H7

FRONT

Sp6

INSIDE

SIDE

Pruritis (Itching)

If pruritis is accompanied by a rash then medical advice' should be sought. Acupressure offers a useful approach in treating itching in a general fashion but if there is an underlying cause then a doctor's advice should lead to identifying and appropriately treating this.

Points:
LiII, Sp10, Sp6 + ear point.

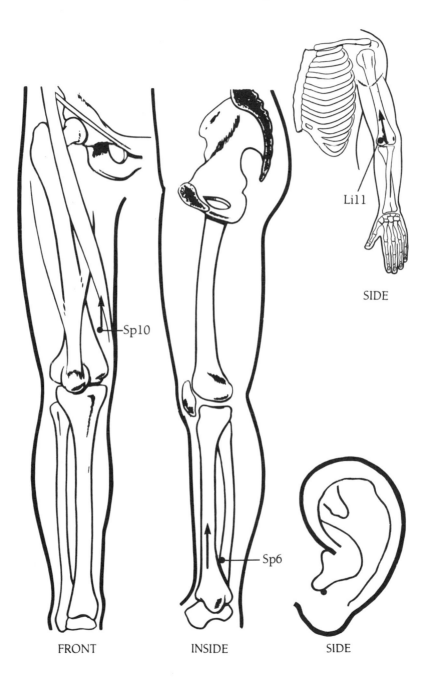

= direction of acupressure massage

Li11

SIDE

Sp10

Sp6

FRONT INSIDE SIDE

9. SPORTS INJURIES

Many more people of all ages are participating in one sport or another, with a resultant increase in the number of sports injuries. From a treatment point of view the most important thing is to treat an injury early.

Acupressure offers an ideal means of doing this. Clearly it is impossible to have a doctor or physiotherapist available at every sporting event, but the average sportsman will be well able to read and understand this book and use acupressure competently. **If you are in any doubt whatsoever about the seriousness of the injury, then appropriate medical advice must be sought.** Remember that in any injury situation there is a possibility of fracture. Acupressure is not a satisfactory or acceptable method of treating a fracture. Commonly sports injuries involve bruising of various degrees of severity, partial or complete muscle tears, tendon injuries and tendon inflammation (tenosynovitis). Acupressure is an effective method of treating all these conditions, except total tendon rupture, most commonly occurring at the Achilles tendon on the ankle.

As well as using acupressure, other measures are important, particularly resting the injured part, and the use of ice packs which cool the tissues and reduce bleeding if any is present. When the initial injury period is passed and the bleeding has stopped then acupressure will come into its own. Where bleeding is present then compression produced by firmly bandaging the affected part serves to limit further bleeding. However, do not bandage so tightly that you stop blood flow altogether. If the fingers or toes of the bandaged limb begin to turn blue then this is a sure sign that compression is too tight and the bandages should be released a little. Elevation of the affected part is also helpful so as to reduce tissue swelling caused as a result of the injury.

If acupressure is used with skill then in many cases the tissue swelling (known as oedema) will often disappear within minutes. In practice this means that the sports injury is dealt with more effectively, and therefore recovery time is shortened. This means that the player will be able to return to his sports activity sooner than he would otherwise have been able to.

ARM INJURIES

Shoulder Joint

This is a common injury and should be treated vigorously. If shoulder pain is left for more than a month then a frozen shoulder may ensue in which stiffness of the joint as well as pain is a troublesome feature. In a chronically painful shoulder which is also stiff, physiotherapy is an essential approach to treatment. Acupressure is usually effective in treatment of the pain.

Points:
Li15, T14, Li11, G21, S38, B57 plus ear point.
Recovery from a true frozen shoulder may take several months.

• Rehabilitation:

1. Even if the shoulder is very painful, it is possible to keep it mobile. Stand facing the back of a chair, leaning on the unaffected arm, and gently rotate the affected arm in ever increasing circles.
2. In a standing position, put the hands together and use the good arm to help the other above the head.
3. In spite of being in pain try to continue performing everyday activities.

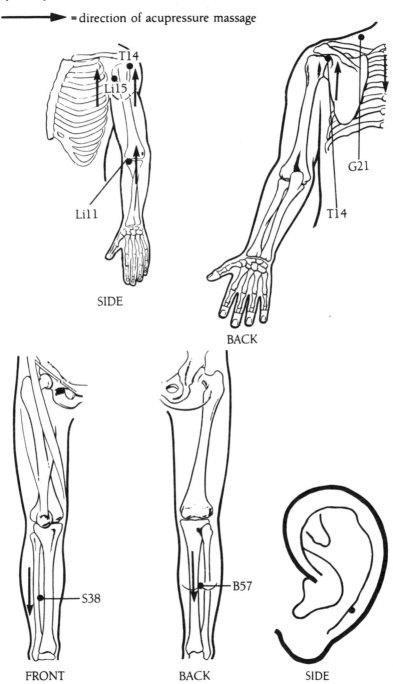

= direction of acupressure massage

T14

Li15

Li11

SIDE

G21

T14

BACK

S38

FRONT

B57

BACK

SIDE

Sterno-clavicular Pain

The sterno-clavicular joint is situated at the inner end of the collar bone, between the collar bone and the breast bone. Sterno-clavicular pain is often aggravated by a fall onto the out-stretched hand and acupressure is an effective way of treating this form of pain.

Points:
Ah Shi (local tender points) plus ear point.

● Rehabilitation:
1. It is possible to keep even a very painful shoulder mobile. Stand facing the back of a chair, leaning on the unaffected arm, and gently rotate the affected arm in ever increasing circles.
2. In a standing position, put the hands together and use the good arm to help the other above the head.
3. In spite of being in pain try to continue performing everyday activities.

→ = direction of acupressure massage

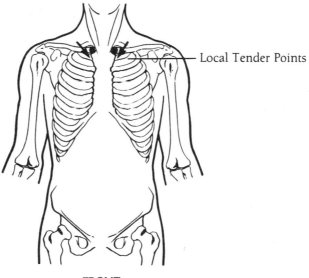

Local Tender Points

FRONT

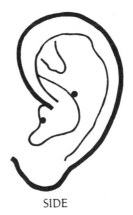

SIDE

Painful Arc (Specific Form of Shoulder Pain)

This is a condition which gives pain when the arm is brought right up above the head. During the middle part of this movement pain is felt in the painful arc syndrome. It's either due to inflammation in one of the tendons around the head of the humerus or due to inflammation in the bursa situated just beneath the acromion, lying between the acromion and the head of the humerus.

Points:
Ah Shi points (local tender points) and Li4 plus ear point.

● Rehabilitation:
Allow 6 weeks for recovery.

It is important to maintain shoulder mobility even though the pain may limit everyday activity.

1. Sit at a polished table with the arm resting on a dry cloth. Keep the arm straight and move the cloth from side to side.

2. Lie on your back with both hands closed together in your lap. Take both hands up and over your head and return.

3. Lie on your back with both arms at your side. Take the injured limb out to the side and then above the head.

= direction of acupressure massage

Local Tender Points —

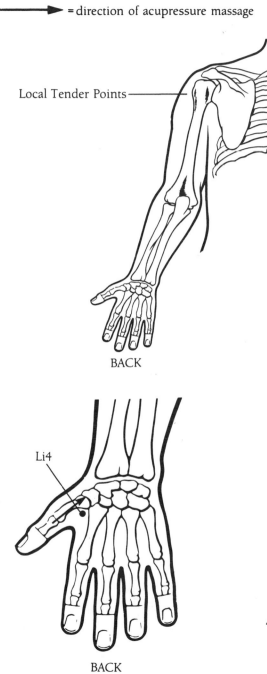

BACK

Li4

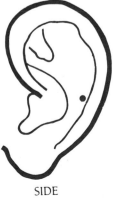

BACK   SIDE

Biceps Tendinitis (Inflammation of Biceps Tendon)

This gives pain along the front of the shoulder joint where the long head of the biceps lies. The injury is common in sports which require vigorous shoulder rotation such as throwing or swimming. Pain is most commonly felt when the arm is reaching in a backwards direction.

Points:
Ah Shi points (local tender points), T5, Li4 plus ear point.

• Rehabilitation:
Allow 3-4 weeks for recovery.

It is important to cease the activity which is causing the pain.

As the pain subsides exercises may commence. To perform these movements keep the arm straight.

1. Swing the arm forwards and backwards, gradually increasing the range of movement.

2. Lie on your back with arms by your side. Take the injured arm up and over your head. Try to press the arm into the floor and return to start position.

→ = direction of acupressure massage

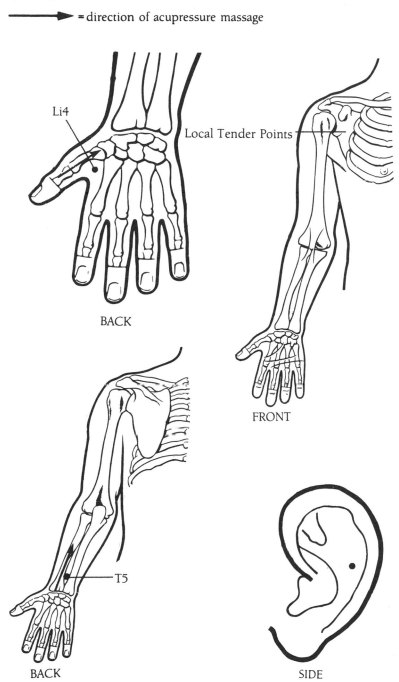

Li4

Local Tender Points

BACK

FRONT

T5

BACK

SIDE

Tennis Elbow

This is usually an over-use injury in which the origin of the extensor muscles situated in the back of the forearm are overstretched and become inflamed. Pain is felt on the outer side of the elbow on gripping, lifting or controlling any heavy object such as a bat or racquet.

Points:
Li11, G34 plus ear point.

● Rehabilitation:
Allow 6 weeks for recovery.

Rest from the activity causing pain and as the condition improves, strengthening exercises may be started.

1. *Improve grip by squeezing the following:*
   (a) ball of wool
   (b) squash ball
   (c) tennis ball

Only when squeezing with (a) is painless may you progress to (b), and so on.

2. *To stretch the muscle insertion:*
Stand facing a wall at a distance of 18 inches. Place the back of the hands on the wall at shoulder height. Bend the arms until the forehead touches the hands and return to the starting position.

3. When pain-free, it is advisable to strengthen the area by wrist-rolling exercises. Stand with your arms in front of you at shoulder height. Hold a towel in the hands. Keeping the arms straight, try to roll the towel into a cylinder.

When returning to racquet games, elbow supports should be used.

= direction of acupressure massage

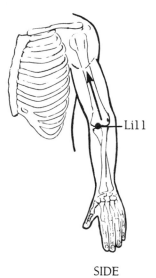

SIDE

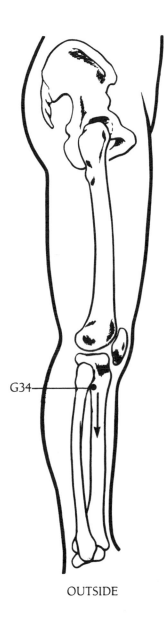

OUTSIDE

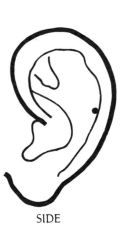

SIDE

Golfer's Elbow

This is a similar condition to tennis elbow but occurring on the inner side of the elbow. It affects the origin of the common flexor muscles situated on the inner aspect of the forearm. Pain is caused by bringing the open palm upwards against resistance and also by forming a grip in certain positions.

Points:
Ah Shi (local tender points), H3 plus ear point.

● Rehabilitation:
Allow 6 weeks for recovery.
To strengthen grip.
1. *Improve grip by squeezing the following:*
    (a) A ball of wool
    (b) A squash ball
    (c) A tennis ball
Only when squeezing with (a) is painless, may you progress to (b), and so on.
2. *To stretch the area:*
Stand 18 inches from a wall. Place the palms of your hands on the wall, fingers inwards. Bend at the elbows until the forehead touches the hands, and return to start position.
3. *To strengthen:*
Sit with the arm resting on the leg, palm facing upwards. Bring the wrist up towards you. To progress, try the exercise while holding a can of food.

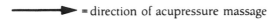 = direction of acupressure massage

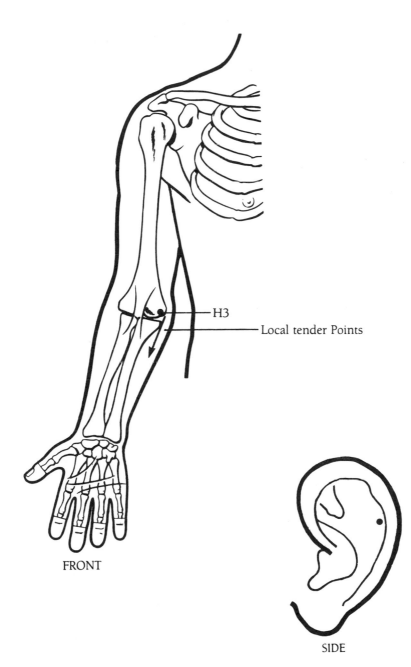

H3

Local tender Points

FRONT

SIDE

Tenosynovitis (Inflammation of Forearm Tendons)

This is inflammation in the extensor muscles, running down the back of the forearm. It is caused by repetitive movements such as rowing, screwdriving etc. The tendon often becomes swollen and feels rough (when the wrist is moved). Rest and strapping with a crepe bandage is required.

Points:
Ah Shi points (local tender points), T5, S36 plus ear point.

• Rehabilitation:
Allow 8-10 weeks for recovery.

When pain and local swelling subside gradually return to exercise - keep the number of repetitions low.

To strengthen grip.

1. *Improve grip by squeezing the following:*
   (a) A ball of wool
   (b) A squash ball
   (c) A tennis ball

Only when squeezing with (a) is painless may you progress to (b), and so on.

2. Sit with the arm resting on the thigh, palm down. Raise the back of the fingers towards the face, keeping the elbow still. To progress, hold a can of food in the hand.

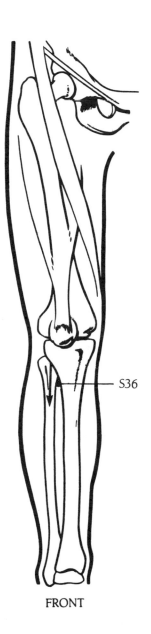

= direction of acupressure massage

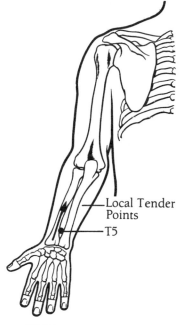

Local Tender Points

T5

BACK

S36

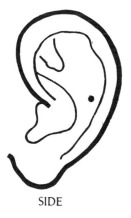

SIDE

FRONT

Wrist Injuries

Wrist sprains are common in contact sports. They are often caused by falls. It is very important to eliminate the possibility of a fracture, particularly an undisplaced Colles fracture of the lower end of the radius.

Points:
Li5, Si5, T4 plus ear point.

• Rehabilitation:
Allow 4-6 weeks for recovery.

1. *To stretch the muscles:*
Stand facing a wall at a distance of 18 inches. Place the back of the hands on the wall at shoulder height. Bend the arms until the forehead touches the hands, and return to the starting position.

2. When pain-free it is advisable to strengthen the area by wrist-rolling exercises. Stand with arm in front of you at shoulder height. Hold a towel in the hands. Keeping the arms straight try to roll the towel into a cylinder.

3. Improve grip by squeezing the following:
   (a) A ball of wool
   (b) A squash ball
   (c) A tennis ball
Only when squeezing with (a) is painless, may you progress to (b) and so on.

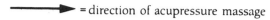 = direction of acupressure massage

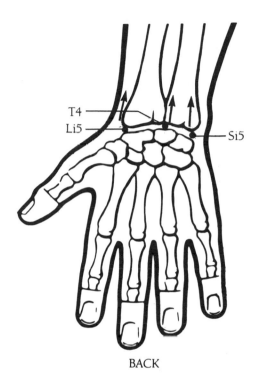

BACK

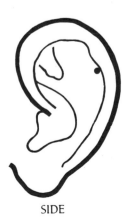

SIDE

Carpal Tunnel Syndrome (Pain and Tingling in the Fingers and Thumb)

Tight arm bands or heavy hand work can sometimes cause a pressure neuritis with typical pain and tingling in the thumb, index, middle and part of the ring finger which is characteristic of carpal tunnel syndrome. Often the fingers feel abnormally large; some patients say that their fingers feel like a bunch of bananas. If there is no improvement after 2 weeks consult your doctor.

Points:
P6, P7 plus ear point.

● Rehabilitation:
When the fingers begin to feel normal the best form of rehabilitation is to use the hand as normally as possible. No specific exercises are required.

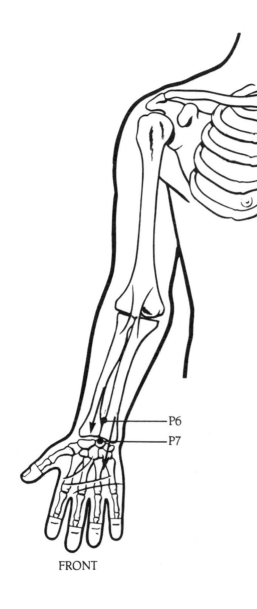

= direction of acupressure massage

P6

P7

FRONT

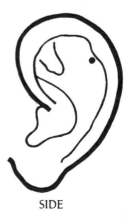

SIDE

Sprained Thumb and Fingers

Sprained thumbs and fingers are common sporting injuries, often caused by the thumb or finger being forced back by contact with another player or during a clumsy basketball catch.

Points:
Ah Shi (local tender points), Li4, Li5 plus ear point.

• Rehabilitation:
Allow 2-3 weeks for recovery.
Wait for 2 days following injury then perform these exercises with the hand in a bowl of hot water:
1. Open and close the fist.
2. Open and close the fingers and thumb.
3. The hand may be immersed in the hot water for 15-20 minutes.
As pain lessens improve grip by squeezing the following:
    (a) A ball of wool
    (b) A squash ball
    (c) A tennis ball
Only when squeezing with (a) is painless, may you progress to (b), and so on.

→ = direction of acupressure massage

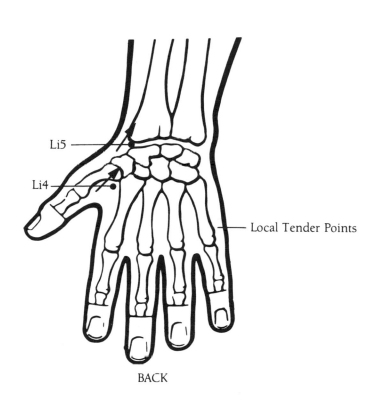

Li5

Li4

Local Tender Points

BACK

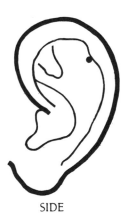

SIDE

SPINAL INJURIES

The spine comprises three areas:

Cervical spine: The neck

Lumbar spine: The lowest quarter of the back

Thoracic spine: The area between the cervical and lumbar spine.

Injuries to the spine fall into distinct categories. One is a direct trauma such as a tackle or fall from a horse. These types of injury must be treated by qualified medical practitioners if the patient is in great pain.

Another category is mechanical problems such as injury when lifting or pushing. Damage may be to muscles, ligaments, or by minor displacement of the vertebrae themselves. Wear and tear due to many factors such as occupation and previous back injuries can also cause spinal problems.

Spinal Injury

Spinal injury is not as common in sport as injury to the limbs. Acute on chronic situation, i.e. back strain on an already chronically bad back, is the most common occurrence.

Neck injuries: Neck injury is most often caused by forceable extension (a backwards movement) of the head. Acupressure can be useful in treating this, but seek out qualified medical opinion.

Points:
G21, Gv14, G20, Si3, Li4, Ah Shi points (local tender points) plus ear point.

• Rehabilitation:
Acute neck injuries often require a surgical collar which removes the weight of the head from the cervical spine.

Exercises are used to regain lost movement. On no account should the neck be forced.

1. Lie on the floor on your back, and turn the head from side to side.

2. Sit in a chair. Try to bring your ear to touch the shoulder. Repeat on both sides.

3. Sit on a chair. Bring your chin to your chest and return to start position.

⟶ = direction of acupressure massage

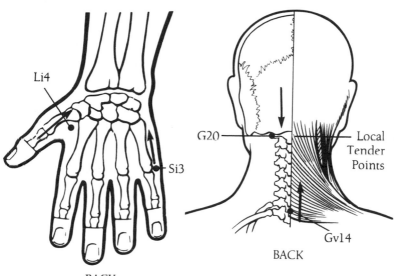

Li4

Si3

G20

Local
Tender
Points

Gv14

BACK

BACK

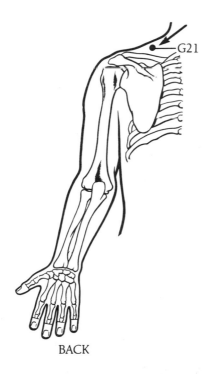

G21

BACK

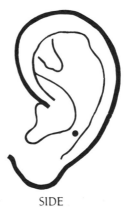

SIDE

Thoracic Spinal Injuries to the Chest Spine

Sometimes injuries are sustained to the middle spine and a number of sportsmen and sportswomen have facet joint problems. These are the small joints at the back of each vertebra. Acupressure is an excellent method of treating this problem.

Points:
Local tender points (Ah Shi points) are shown in the diagram B12 to B19 depending on the site of the pain, plus ear point.

• Rehabilitation:
1. Lie face down with the hands behind the neck. Raise the head and shoulders as high as you can and return.
2. Sit in a chair. Reach from side to side towards the floor with each hand in turn.
3. Sit on the edge of a chair and turn around to look behind you. Repeat to the other side.

⟶ = direction of acupressure massage

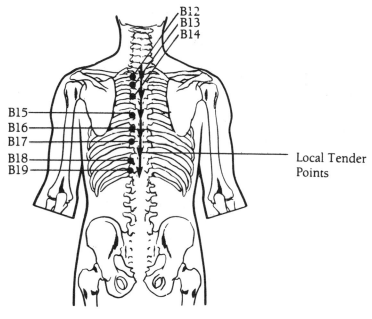

BACK

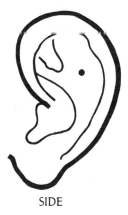

SIDE

Lumbar Spine

Most commonly there is a predisposing cause such as narrow discs in the lower lumbar spine. Discs lie between the vertebrae and cushion one vertebra from the next. If the condition does not respond satisfactorily to treatment with acupressure then qualified medical opinion should be sought. In most cases it is essential to try conservative measures first. Acupressure is well worth a try and is often successful for relieving low back pain.

Points:
B31, B25, B40, G30, Ah Shi points (local tender points) plus ear point.

● Rehabilitation:
Allow 4 weeks for recovery.
1. Lie face downwards with the hands behind the back. Lift the head and shoulders off the floor.
2. Lie on your back with knees bent, feet on the floor. Move both legs from side to side.
3. When pain-free, stand with hands clasped behind the back, and move the upper body forwards and backwards, gradually increasing the amount of movement.

→ = direction of acupressure massage

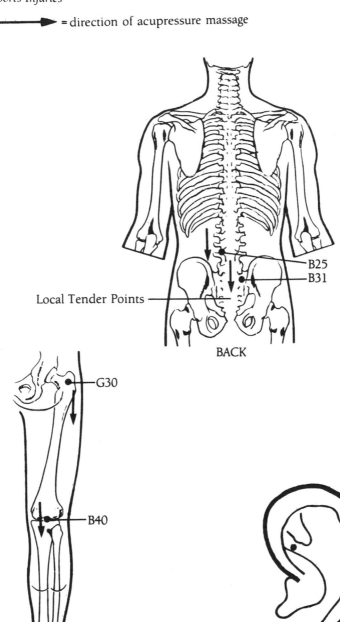

B25
B31

Local Tender Points

BACK

G30

B40

BACK

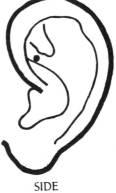

SIDE

TRUNK INJURIES

Rib Injuries

Bruised, cracked or fractured ribs are common in contact sport and characteristically cause pain which is aggravated by deep breathing. Modern treatment does not favour local strapping of the ribs, and therefore some treatment for the pain is essential in order to enable normal breathing to take place. Occasionally rib pain may be caused by the muscles between the ribs being strained. Acupressure is ideal for this.

Points:

G34, Liv3 plus Ah Shi points (local tender points B12 to B19); plus ear point.

• Rehabilitation:

Undisplaced rib fractures may take 4-6 weeks for recovery. When rib fractures are healed or as the pain subsides lie on your back with the arms by the side. Take the arms up and over the head. At the same time breathe in until discomfort is felt or the lungs are completely filled.

Stand with arms crossed in front of you, take one arm up and out to the side and continue the movement as far as it will go. Return to start position and repeat with the other arm.

→ = direction of acupressure massage

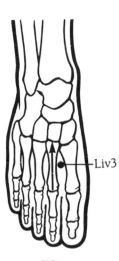

TOP

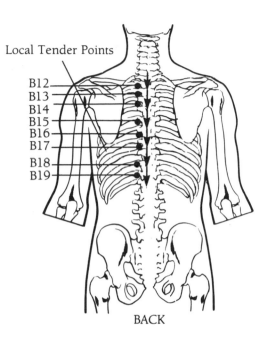

Local Tender Points

B12
B13
B14
B15
B16
B17
B18
B19

—Liv3

BACK

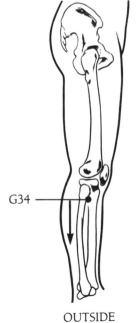

G34 —

OUTSIDE

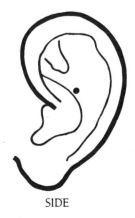

SIDE

Stitch

This is a cramp-like muscular pain which occurs in the lower part of the abdomen. It comes on after exercise. Any lower abdominal pain which persists after rest requires a medical opinion. Some people are especially liable to stitch, and in these cases acupressure is of use.

Points:
Sp6, S36, Cv6, Ah Shi points (local tender points) plus ear point.

• Rehabilitation:
Allow 3–4 weeks for recovery as the pain subsides.
Try the following
Starting position is lying on your back on the floor with knees bent, feet flat on the floor.

Raise only your head off the floor.

Head and shoulders raise.

Reach with the hands to touch the knees.

Arms folded across the chest, sit up to touch the elbows to the knees.

———▶ = direction of acupressure massage

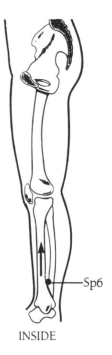

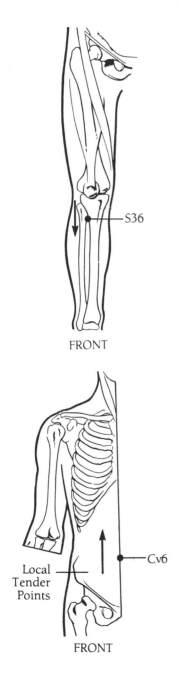

FRONT

INSIDE

FRONT

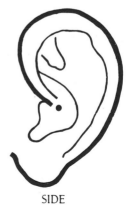

SIDE

GROIN AND HIP INJURIES

The group of muscles in the groin is situated on the inner aspect of the thigh. Injury may occur when an unintentional splits movement takes places such as on muddy or slippery surfaces. Kicking or tackling movements with the inside of the foot and sudden twisting or turning movements can also cause injury. Pain may also be felt higher in the groin, to the ilio-psoas muscle, due to repetition of the kicking action. If this movement is stopped, the injury usually clears up in 2 or 3 weeks.

Adductor Pain (Pain on Inside of Thigh)

If the legs are forced apart during a sports injury, this often strains the adductor ligament which is situated right at the top of the inside of the thigh. Acupressure can be useful in treating this problem.

Points:
Ah Shi points (local tender points) plus ear point.

• Rehabilitation:
Allow 6 weeks for recovery.

It is important to stretch this muscle injury in order to prevent further injury upon return to sport activities.

1. Sit on the floor with the legs apart. Try to reach as far forward as you can.

2. Stand with legs wide apart. Touch the floor as far in front and behind you as possible.

3. Stand with the legs wide apart and attempt to move the feet further apart.

4. Improve the muscle power by squeezing a pillow or football between the knees. Hold the position for 10 seconds each time.

5. In the later stages of ,recovery, breaststroke swimming is recommended for strengthening the muscles.

→ = direction of acupressure massage

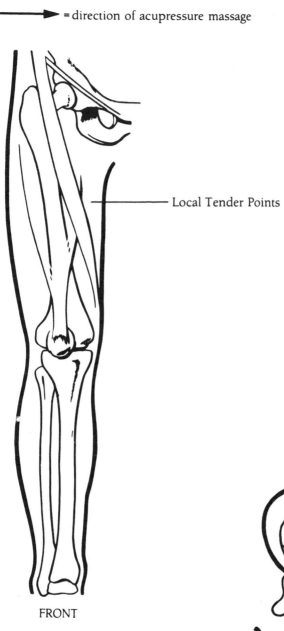

Local Tender Points

FRONT

SIDE

Abdominal Strain (Pain in the Rectus Abdominis Muscle)

The rectus abdominis are a pair of muscles lying in the wall of the abdomen, passing from the pelvis up to the front part of the lower edge of the rib cage. These muscles are often strained. This may be due to over-use in training in some cases, or to a direct blow.

Injury may occur during violent movement such as in a judo fall, or by lifting heavy objects. Multiple sit-ups performed too quickly or too powerfully can also cause problems.

Points:
Sp6, S36, Cv6, Ah Shi points (local tender points) plus ear point.

• Rehabilitation:
Allow 3-4 weeks for recovery as the pain subsides.

Try the following exercises. The starting position is lying on your back, on the floor with knees bent, feet flat on the floor:

1. Raise only your head off the floor.
2. Raise head and shoulders.
3. Reach with the hands to touch the knees.
4. With arms folded across the chest, sit up and touch the elbows to the knees.

——————▶ = direction of acupressure massage

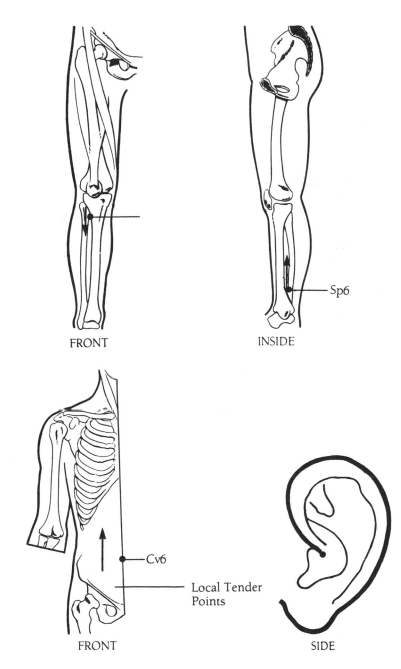

FRONT

INSIDE

Sp6

FRONT

Cv6

Local Tender
Points

SIDE

Hip Injuries

The hip is a strong joint and is not often injured during sport. However, the outer aspect of the thigh at the level of the hip is sometimes injured by direct contact with the ground or another player, causing various degrees of bruising.

Recovery from bruising may take 2 weeks.

Points:
Ah Shi points (local tender points), G29, S31, G30, G34, plus ear point.

• Rehabilitation:
Maintaining the range of movement of the hips is vital.

1. Lie face down and lift one leg at a time, keeping the leg straight.

2. Lie on the side of the uninjured leg. Lift the injured leg as high as possible, keeping it straight.

3. Lie on your back, and bring the knee up to the chest.

4. Sit on the floor, keep the legs straight and turn the feet inwards and outwards.

5. When pain subsides, swimming is recommended.

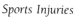 = direction of acupressure massage

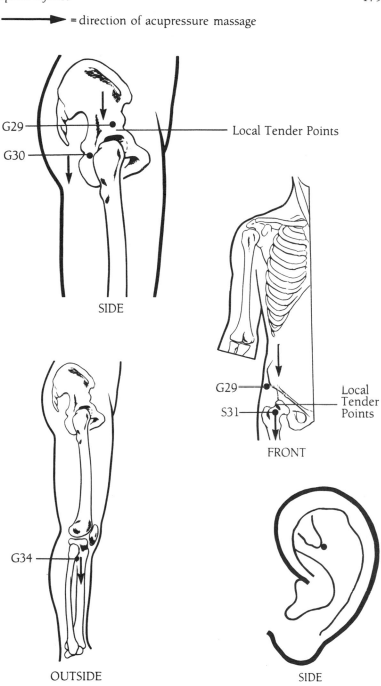

G29 — Local Tender Points

G30

SIDE

G29 — Local Tender Points

S31

FRONT

G34

OUTSIDE

SIDE

THIGH INJURIES

Deadleg

Any muscle may receive a direct blow thereby causing temporary stiffness with pain. The term deadleg is reserved for the muscles on the front and side of the thigh. The direct blow will cause internal bleeding with resultant swelling, pain and loss of function.

Points:
Ah Shi (local tender points), G34, G44, plus ear point.

● Rehabilitation:
1-2 weeks may be required for full recovery.

The quadriceps muscle in front of the thigh will soon become weak and therefore the exercises given for knee injuries (see page 188) should be followed.

When this sequence of exercises has been completed successfully, cycling and swimming are recommended.

Return to sport is dependent upon full pain-free movement at the knee and hip joints.

= direction of acupressure massage

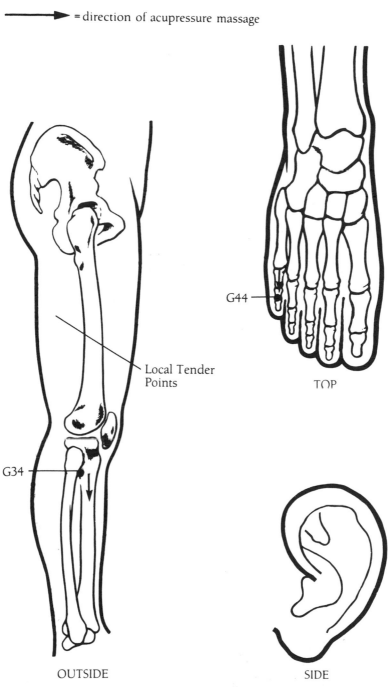

Local Tender
Points

G44

TOP

G34

OUTSIDE

SIDE

Rectus Femoris

This muscle lies on the front of the thigh running from the front of the hip to the knee. It is injured mainly during sprinting and kicking.

Points:
Ah Shi (local tender points) G34, plus ear point.

• Rehabilitation
Allow 4–6 weeks for recovery.
Static Exercise
1. Sit on the floor, keeping the injured leg straight and tighten the muscles of the thigh. When this is done correctly, the heel will lift just clear of the floor (compared with the other leg). Hold the position for 10 seconds each time.
2. Sit on the floor and place a pillow or rolled towel behind the knee. Tighten the thigh muscles and raise the heel from the floor.
3. Sit on a table. Straighten and bend the leg.
4. Stand leaning on a table, and bend both knees just a few degrees. Increase movement as confidence returns.

Stretching
In the early stages of rehabilitation, begin by kneeling on the floor with the trunk upright. As the pain diminishes, gradually lean backwards using the hands to support the body weight. The eventual aim is to bring the back of the head as near as possible to the floor.

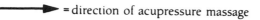 = direction of acupressure massage

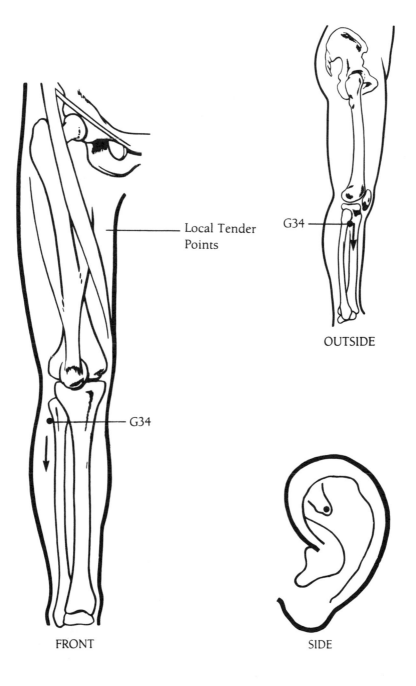

Local Tender
Points

G34

OUTSIDE

G34

FRONT

SIDE

Hamstring

This group of muscles lies on the back of the thigh. They affect the movement of both the hip and the knee joints. These muscles are frequently injured in sport during fast movements such as sprinting. Injury also occurs due to overstretching, as when kicking a ball.

Lack of warm-up and fatigue are other possible causes, as are uncoordinated movements and occasionally direct violence – for example, receiving a kick from behind.

Points:
Ah Shi points (local tender points) B40 plus ear point.

● Rehabilitation:
It is very important to maintain or even improve the amount of stretch in the hamstrings following injury:
1. Sit on the floor with both legs straight, and raise the injured leg until discomfort is felt. Ease of movement will improve each day.
2. Sit on the floor with the injured leg straight and the other leg bent. Reach forward with the hands to touch the toes. If this is achieved easily, reach beyond the toes.
3. Stand, keeping the legs straight, and reach to the floor. Aim to improve each day.
4. Stand on the uninjured leg with the injured leg resting on an object parallel with the floor. Reach towards the foot of the injured leg.

➡ = direction of acupressure massage

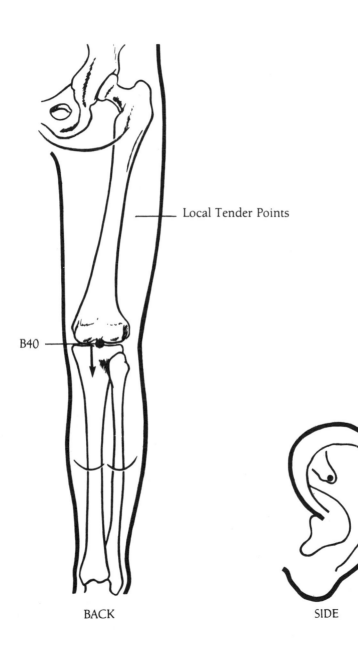

Local Tender Points

B40

BACK

SIDE

KNEE AND LOWER LEG INJURIES

Cartilages

These are usually damaged because of a violent movement of the knee while the foot is stationary, such as twisting when wearing soccer boots with studs.

The injury causes locking, giving way, swelling and pain. Only one of these symptoms may be felt, although in some cases all of them are. When this happens qualified medical help should be sought.

Ligaments

These are situated on the inner (medial ligament) and outer (lateral ligament) aspects of the joint. These prevent excessive sideways movement. Inside the joint are the cruciate ligaments which prevent excessive forward and backward movement.

Ligaments are injured when the joint is forced into unnatural positions such as a block tackle. At the front of the knee is the ligamentum patellae which attaches the knee cap to the front of the tibia.

Points:

Xiyan (the so called eyes of the knee) Sp9, B40 plus ear point. Ligament strains may take 6 weeks for recovery.

● Rehabilitation:

It is vital to maintain the size and strength of the quadriceps muscle (on the front of the thigh from hip to knee). These exercises should be performed in sequence, moving on to the next exercise only when pain subsides.

Static Exercise

1. Sit on the floor, keeping the leg straight. Tighten the muscles of the thigh. When this is done correctly the heel will lift just clear of the floor (compare with the other leg). Hold the position for 10 seconds each time.
2. Sit on the floor and place a pillow or rolled towel behind the knee. Tighten the thigh muscles and raise the heel from the floor.
3. Sit on a table. Straighten and bend the leg.
4. Stand leaning on a table, and bend both knees, just a few degrees. Increase movement as confidence returns.
5. Stand in front of a kitchen chair, bend the knees until your buttocks touch the seat, and return to the start position.

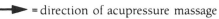 = direction of acupressure massage

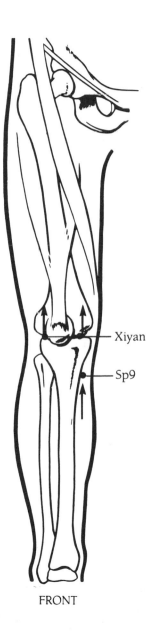

Xiyan

Sp9

FRONT

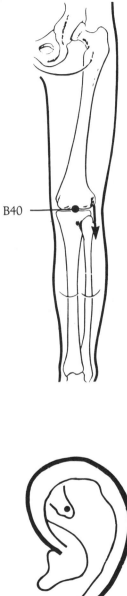

B40

SIDE

Lateral Ligament Strain (Pain on the Outer side of the Knee Joint)

Injury occurs when strain is put onto the outside of the joint, such as in a tackle or when, in basketball, a player lands on the outer side of the foot.

Points:
Ah Shi (local tender points) plus ear point.

● Rehabilitation:
It is vital to maintain the size and strength of the quadriceps muscle (on the front of the thigh from hip to knee).

These exercises should be performed in sequence, moving on to the next exercise only when pain subsides.

Static Exercise

1. Sit on the floor, keeping the leg straight. Tighten the muscles of the thigh. When this is done correctly, the heel will lift just clear of the floor (compare with the other leg). Hold the position for 10 seconds each time.

2. Sit on the floor and place a pillow or rolled towel behind the knee. Tighten the thigh muscles and raise the heel from the floor.

3. Sit on a table. Straighten and bend the leg.

4. Stand leaning on a table, and bend both knees just a few degrees. Increase movement as confidence returns.

5. Stand in front of a kitchen chair, bend the knees until your buttocks touch the seat, and return to the start position.

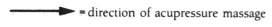 = direction of acupressure massage

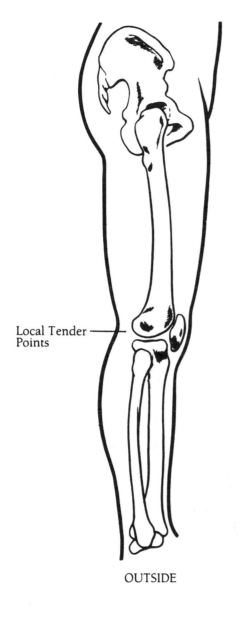

Local Tender Points

OUTSIDE

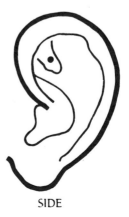

SIDE

Medial Ligament Sprain (Sprain of Ligament on Inner Side of Knee)

This is perhaps the most common sporting injury of the knee, because the ligament on the inside of the knee (known as the medial ligament of the knee) is particularly vulnerable to rotation of the leg about a fixed foot such as may occur during football or skiing. Severe cases of these injuries may also produce tearing of the cartilages in the knee joint.

Points:
Ah Shi points (local tender points) plus ear point.

● Rehabilitation:
It is vital to maintain the size and strength of the quadriceps muscle (on the front of the thigh from hip to knee).

These exercises should be performed in sequence, moving on to the next exercise only when pain subsides.

Static Exercise

1. Sit on the floor, keeping the leg straight. Tighten the muscles of the thigh. When this is done correctly the heel will lift just clear of the floor (compare with the other leg). Hold the position for 10 seconds each time.
2. Sit on the floor and place a pillow or rolled towel behind the knee. Tighten the thigh muscles and raise the heel from the floor.
3. Sit on a table. Straighten and bend the leg.
4. Stand leaning on a table, and bend both knees just a few degrees. Increase movement as confidence returns.
5. Stand in front of a kitchen chair, bend the knees until your buttocks touch the seat, and return to the start position.

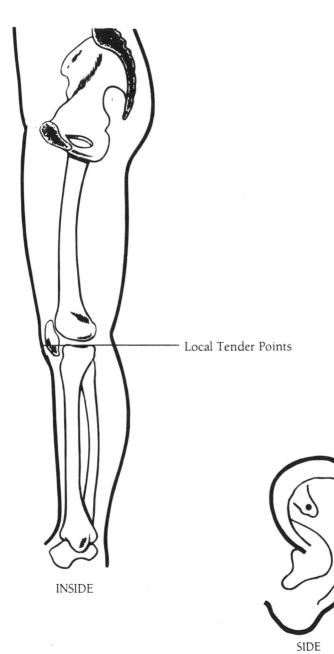

= direction of acupressure massage

Local Tender Points

INSIDE

SIDE

Lower Leg Injuries

Injuries to the lower leg are very common and are suffered particularly by long-distance runners, aerobics teachers, and athletes who change the surface which they train and compete on too often. If the problem will not clear up, seek qualified medical help to remove the possibility of stress fractures and Anterior Tibial Syndrome.

Shin Soreness

Sometimes known as shin splints this injury is common in runners. It produces pain on or next to the tibia (the major bone in the lower leg) during active weight bearing.

Points:
Ah Shi points (local tender points) Sp9 plus ear point.

• Rehabilitation:
Allow 6–8 weeks for recovery.
   Rest from the offending form of exercise.
   The use of shock-absorbing inner soles is recommended.

= direction of acupressure massage

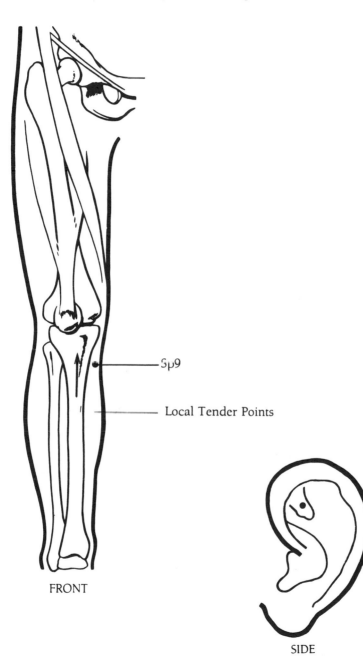

Sp9

Local Tender Points

FRONT

SIDE

Calf Strains

The calf muscles lie in the back of the lower leg. There are two main muscles, the gastrocnemius and the soleus muscles. They both insert into the achilles tendon which attaches to the heel bone. Muscle injury may be caused by fatigue; for example, because of insufficient warming-up or during the closing minutes of a strenuous game. Sudden changes of direction, such as in tennis and squash, may also lead to injury, as will direct violence such as a kick.

Points:
B40, B57, Ah Shi (local tender points) plus ear point.

• Rehabilitation:
These exercises should be done in the following sequence as pain subsides.
1. Lie on a sofa or on the floor with the legs elevated (feet above the hips). Push the toes away from you and return.
2. Sit in a chair with the feet flat on the floor, raise the heels and return to the starting position.
3. Lean on a table, raise yourself up on to your toes and return to the starting position. Take the weight with the arms.
4. Stand and rise up and down on your toes.
5. Stand and rise up and down on the toes of one foot.

Stretching Exercise
Face a wall and lean against it with both hands. Walk slowly away from the wall, keeping the hands in position. Try to keep the heels pressed down all the time.

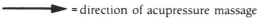 = direction of acupressure massage

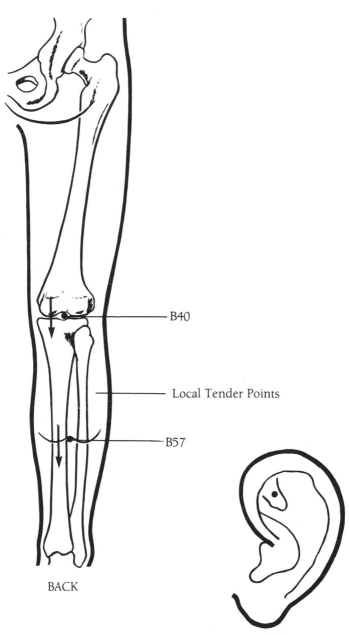

B40

Local Tender Points

B57

BACK

SIDE

Achilles Tendinitis (Inflammation of Achilles Tendon)

In this condition pain is felt in the achilles tendon just above the heel. The tendon is often painful to touch. Rupture of the achilles tendon is uncommon. However, if the tendon is partially or completely ruptured, acupressure is not a suitable method of therapy and competent orthopaedic treatment should be sought.

Points:
Ah Shi points (local tender points) plus ear point.

● Rehabilitation:
These exercises should be done in the following sequence as pain subsides.
1. Lie on a sofa or on the floor with the legs elevated (feet above the hips). Push the toes away from you and return.
2. Sit in a chair with the feet flat on the floor, raise the heels and return to the starting position.
3. Lean on a table, raise yourself up on to your toes and return to the starting position. Take the weight with the arms.
4. Stand and rise up and down on your toes.
5. Stand and rise up and down on the toes of one foot.

Stretching Exercise
Face a wall and lean against it with both hands. Walk slowly away from the wall, keeping the hands in position. Try to keep the heels pressed down all the time.

⟶ = direction of acupressure massage

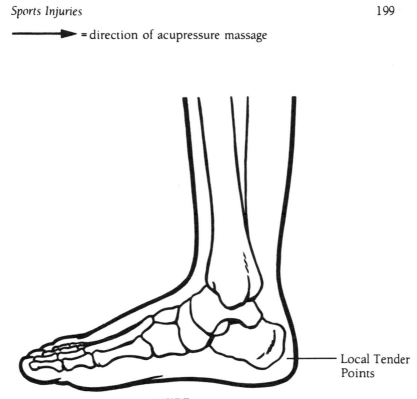

Local Tender Points

INSIDE

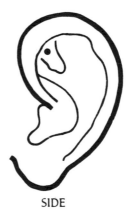

SIDE

Leg Cramp

The commonest causes of leg cramps are tight fitting garments such as socks with elastic around the tops, fatigue or unaccustomed muscle strain, or salt deficiency and dehydration. If a tight fitting garment is worn, loosen it. If salt deficiency and dehydration is present drink a solution of salt in water. In fatigue or unaccustomed muscle strain use acupressure.

Points:

B40, B57, Ah Shi points (local tender points) plus ear point. Cramp elsewhere in the body should be treated by using local tender points.

= direction of acupressure massage

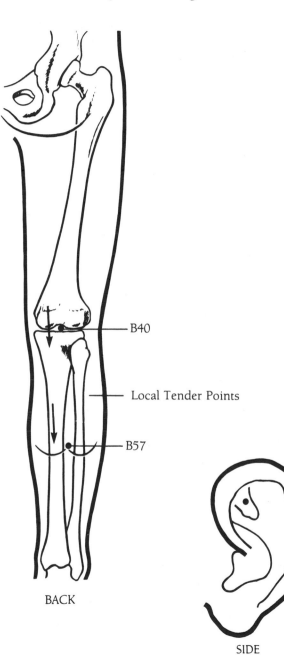

B40

Local Tender Points

B57

BACK

SIDE

Ankle Injuries

Ankle sprains are often caused by a forced sideways movement to the inside or the outside of the ankle. The ligaments on each side of the joint capsule may be stretched or torn and may bleed internally or externally.

Points:
S41, Sp5, G40 plus ear point.

• Rehabilitation:
The following exercises should be done in sequence as pain diminishes.
1. Sit with the leg elevated.
  (a) Push your toes away from you and bring them towards you.
  (b) Turn the foot inwards and outwards.
  (c) Draw circles with the foot.
2. Sit on a chair, feet flat on the floor, and raise the heels off the floor. Return to the starting position.
3. Stand, leaning on a table. Raise the heels off the floor and return.
4. Stand, raise the heels off the floor and return.

Balance
Ankle injuries cause a temporary loss of balance and reorientation is therefore required.
1. Stand on the injured leg only and try to remain in this position for 1 minute. When you have managed this, close your eyes and try again.
2. Stand on the toes of the injured leg and try to remain in this position for 30 seconds.

→ = direction of acupressure massage

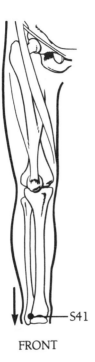

S41

FRONT

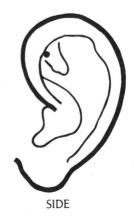

Sp5

INSIDE

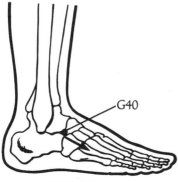

G40

OUTSIDE

SIDE

FOOT INJURIES

Bruised Heel

Pain beneath the heel is often due to simple bruising, which may happen when landing during jumping or hurdling.

Points:
Ah Shi points (local tender points) plus ear point.

• Rehabilitation:
Refrain from the sport or exercise causing the injury.

The use of shock-absorbing heel inserts is recommended in all shoes worn.

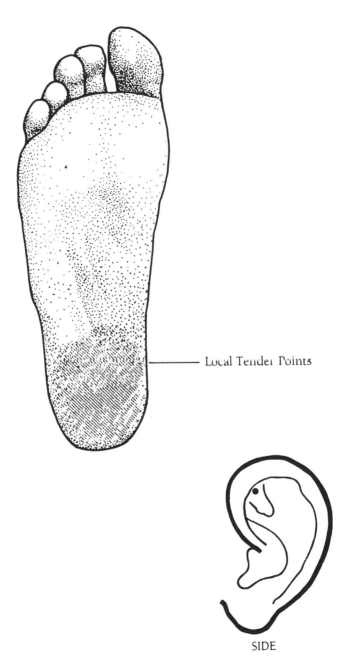

= direction of acupressure massage

Local Tender Points

SIDE

Plantar Fascitis (Pain on Sole of Foot)

In this condition pain is felt on the sole of the foot, in front of the bone under the heel. It is called inflammation of the plantar fascia, which is a very thick band of fibrous tissue connecting the heel to the metatarsal arch at the front of the foot. It occurs mostly in those sports involving running or treading on hard surfaces. Acupressure is very useful in treating this condition. The method of treating plantar fascitis is exactly the same as for treating foot strain, which is a commoner sporting injury.

Points:
Ah Shi points (local tender points) plus ear point.

● Rehabilitation:
Refrain from the sport or exercise causing the problem.

The use of shock-absorbing inner soles is recommended.

Use foam rubber to build up additional support for the arch of the foot.

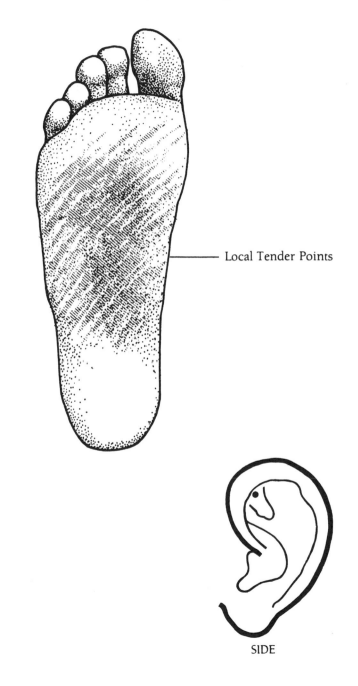

➤ = direction of acupressure massage

Local Tender Points

SIDE

Metatarsalgia (Pain on Ball of Foot)

This is pain under the ball of the foot where the supporting ligaments of the metatarsal heads become strained in the line of the toe joints. It is a common complaint among those who stand a lot at work and is also caused by running or jumping on hard surfaces, or running in hard-soled shoes. Appropriate foot wear is essential in these cases, and metatarsal support is mandatory.

Points:
Extra points plus Ah Shi points (local tender points) plus ear point.

• Rehabilitation:
Refrain from the sport or exercise causing the problem.

The use of shock-absorbing inner soles is recommended.

A metatarsal bar of foam rubber or felt may also assist in relieving the pain. This can be purchased from a chemist or chiropodist.

→ = direction of acupressure massage

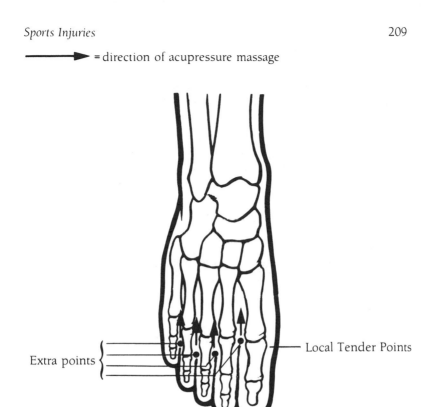

Extra points

Local Tender Points

TOP

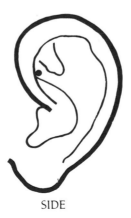

SIDE

Hallux Valgus (Pain on Bunion Joint of Foot)

This is pain in the big toe joint and is common in older sportsmen. Excessive use of tight foot wear over the years causes bunions, which are swellings of the joint at the base of the big toe. This swelling is often followed by diversion of the joint from its original straight lines towards the outer side of the foot, the characteristic deformity of hallux valgus.

Points:
Liv3, Ah Shi points (local tender points) plus ear point.

• Rehabilitation:
Shock-absorbing inner soles are recommended in all shoes worn.

= direction of acupressure massage

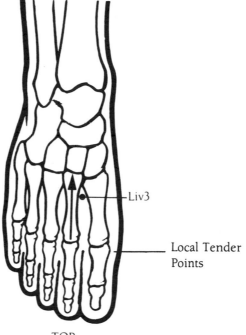

Liv3

Local Tender
Points

TOP

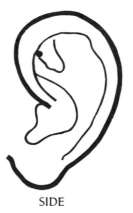

SIDE

FURTHER READING

If you want to learn more about acupuncture, there are a number of books available, of which the following is a selection.

Textbooks on Traditional Chinese Acupuncture

Modern Chinese Acupuncture by G.T. and N.R. Lewith, published by Thorsons.

The Acupuncture Treatment of Internal Disease by G.T. Lewith, published by Thorsons.

Modern Techniques of Acupuncture

Modern Techniques of Acupuncture, Volumes I, II and III by Dr Julian Kenyon, published by Thorsons.

Acupuncture Without Needles

The electro stimulation of Energy Points for the relief of pain and the treatment of other conditions, by Dr Julian Kenyon M.D., M.B., Ch.B. (Available only from Auto-Compute Trading Ltd., Suite 1B, Market Centre, Western International Market, Hayes Road, Southall, Middlesex UB2 5XJ, England.)

Books on Sports Medicine

Sport and Medicine by Peter N. Sperryn, published by Butterworths,

Sports Injuries, a Self Help Guide by Vivian Grisogono, published by John Murray.

USEFUL ADDRESSES

U.K.
British Medical Acupuncture Society, 77-79 Chancery Lane, London WC2.

United States
Acupuncture International Association, 2330 S. Brentwood Boulevard, St. Louis, MO 63144.

Canada
Acupuncture Foundation for Canada, 10 St Mary Street, Toronto ON M4Y1P9.

Australia
Arthritis and Rheumatism Council, Wynward House, 291 George Street, Sydney NSW 2000.
Australian Arthritis and Rheumatism Foundation, The Queen Elizabeth Hospital, Woodville, South Australia 5011.

New Zealand
Arthritis and Rheumatism Foundation of New Zealand, P.O. Box 10-020 Southern Cross Building, Brandon Street, Wellington.
New Zealand Medical Acupuncture Society, P.O. Box 37-025, Parnell, Auckland, New Zealand.

South Africa
South Africa Rheumatism and Arthritis Association, Namaqua House, 26 Burg Street, Cape Town 8001.
South African National Acupuncture Association, Box 2172, Johannesburg 2000, South Africa.

INDEX